Diseases of the Mouth, Lips, Tongue, Teeth & Gums

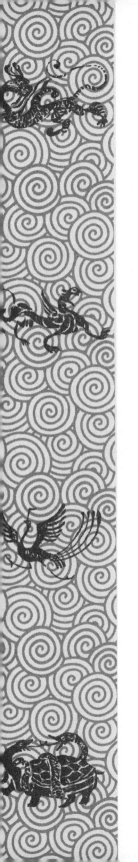

The Treatment of Disease in TCM

VOLUME 3:

Diseases of the Mouth, Lips, Tongue, Teeth & Gums

 by Philippe Sionneau
& Lü Gang

BLUE POPPY PRESS

Published by:

BLUE POPPY PRESS, INC.
1775 LINDEN AVE.
BOULDER, CO 80304

First Edition, January, 1997

ISBN 0-936185-79-1
LC 91-83249

COMP Designation: Original work using a standard translational terminology

Printed at Johnson Printing on recycled, elementally chlorine-free paper

10 9 8 7 6 5 4 3 2 1

The author may be reached at the following address:
Philippe Sionneau
54, rue de Wattignies
75012 Paris, France

Author's Foreword

Most TCM textbooks and clinical handbooks describe the diagnosis and treatment of the same major diseases and conditions. These can be either traditional Chinese disease categories, such as lateral costal pain, *shan* qi, and the strangury and turbidity, or they may be modern Western disease diagnoses, such as cholecystitis, chronic appendicitis, Bell's palsy, and endometriosis. However, patients coming to Western acupuncturists or practitioners of Chinese medicine often complain of unpleasant or unusual symptoms which neither modern Western nor contemporary Traditional Chinese Medicine consider diseases in and of themselves. These may include, for instance, dry nose, heavy-headedness, strong smelling armpits, loss of the sense of taste, itchy eyes, coldness in the low back region, tremor of the hands, sweating of the hands, or premature greying of the hair. Thus, these all too commonly encountered complaints do not appear as chapters in our TCM textbooks, and, therefore, we Western practitioners may have trouble finding out about their TCM diagnosis and treatment. Without delving into the Chinese medical literature more deeply, we might even be tempted to say that Chinese medicine does not address many of the complaints of our Western patients.

Being fully aware of this difficulty, when studying in China, I made a special attempt to discover and collect original information on such symptoms or diseases which typically are overlooked in the majority of the literature. My aim was to enlarge our understanding and to widen our knowledge so as to increase our clinical efficacy. This has led me to write the third of this series of practical books for clinical use, classified according to the part of the body where these symptoms appear. These books will cover the main, standard or classical diseases of Chinese medicine as well as a host of other minor diseases and complaints which nonetheless appear often in our real-life patients.

This new approach offers two further advantages besides filling in the gaps in our Western language TCM literature. First, when a patient's major complaint is difficult to diagnose and analyze due to a confused or complicated situation and when a thorough knowledge of the usual methods of diagnosis and of the standard diseases are not sufficient, these nonstandard or little written about symptoms and diseases can help us tackle the problem from a different angle.

For example, if the signs and symptoms of sinusitis or rhinitis in one of our patients do not clearly fall under the usual pattern discrimination of *bi yuan* (deep source nasal congestion), we might find our patient's pattern under dry nose (*bi gan*), nose pain (*bi tong*), itchy nose (*bi yang*), bad odor of the nose (*bi chou*), or acid, sour nose (*bi suan*) if our patient suffers from one of these symptoms. Thus we can approach their case from a slightly different perspective.

The second advantage is that this series of books will offer a new and more exhaustive approach to a number of key symptoms, such as spontaneous perspiration, night sweats, aversion to wind and cold, red cheeks, pale nails, and purple lips. Most current Western language TCM texts only discuss the most basic disease causes and disease mechanisms, patterns and their treatments for these symptoms and conditions, and patients often present with patterns not included in these texts. The causes and mechanisms of these complaints are, in fact, more numerous and varied than most books commonly describe. For example, most books emphasize that night sweats are due to yin vacuity with vacuity heat. But what about heart blood vacuity, spleen vacuity with damp encumbrance, *shao yang* disease, damp heat, and the other causes of night sweats? Or take vexatious heat in the five hearts. It is also typically described as a consequence of yin vacuity and vacuity heat. Whereas, it can just as well be caused by depressive heat in the liver, blood stasis, evils hidden in the yin aspect, heat internally depressed, etc.

Because I am more specialized in internal medicine and Chinese medicinals, I thought it best to ask my friend Lu Gang to compose the acupuncture and moxibustion treatments. When studying in Wuhan, Lu Gang was the person who had the deepest influence on my comprehension of Chinese medicine. He proved to be a competent and efficient guide who helped me reach a more subtle understanding of TCM terminology. Thanks to his outstanding abilities, he obtained a Master of Acupuncture & Moxibustion Degree from the Nanjing College of TCM and has a thorough knowledge of this art. It appeared, therefore, quite logical to ask him to collaborate on this series of books, both in gratitude for the help he has given me in the past and because I was sure his collaboration would enhance the quality of this series.

The terminology in this book is based on Nigel Wiseman's *Glossary of Chinese Medical Terms and Acupuncture Points*, Paradigm Publications, Brookline, MA, 1990 with up-dates and revisions supplied by Nigel Wiseman through Bob Felt of Paradigm Publications. Other divergences from Dr. Wiseman's terminology are noted and discussed in the footnotes.

For further information on the use of processed Chinese medicinals, the reader is referred to my book, *Pao Zhi: An Introduction to the Use of Processed Chinese Medicinals*, also published by Blue Poppy Press. It is my belief that processed medicinals are far more effective than unprocessed medicinals. In TCM, each specific medicinal is identified not only by its species and part or piece but also by its method of processing. Thus, a medicinal consisting of the same part from the same species is a different medicinal if it is processed differently. Obviously, it is extremely important to use the right medicinal in the right situation, and using processed medicinals is, in my opinion, an integral part of using the right medicinal.

All formula dosages are given for a single day's administration unless otherwise stated. In addition, these dosages are for adults. Dosages for children should be adjusted according to their body weight.

Hopefully, this book and the others to come in this series will help Western practitioners to make progress in the universe of TCM for the benefit of suffering people.

Philippe Sionneau
October 30, 1996
Paris, France

Contents

Author's Foreword, v

1   Bland Taste in the Mouth 1

2   Bitter Taste in the Mouth 7

3   Salty Taste in the Mouth 11

4   Sour Taste in the Mouth 15

5   Burning or Peppery Taste in the Mouth 21

6   Sweet Taste in the Mouth 23

7   Sliminess in the Mouth 27

8   Malodorous Mouth 31

9   Oral Thirst 37

10   Drooling from the Corner of the Mouth 53

11   Mouth Sores 61

12   Copious Spittle 65

13   Crimson Lips 69

14   Cyanotic Lips 71

15   Pale White Lips 81

16   Cracked Dry Lips 85

17   Lip Tremor 91

18   Swelling, Itching & Pain in the Lips 95

19   Swollen Tongue 97

20   Fat Tongue 103

21   Trembling Tongue 107

22   Stiff Tongue 115

23   Numbness of the Tongue 121

24   Limp Tongue 127

25   Painful Tongue 135

26 Curled Tongue 145
27 Dry Tongue 149
28 Fissured Tongue 153
29 Spontaneous Bleeding of the Tongue 157
30 Tongue Sores 163
31 Worrying Tongue 171
32 Protracted Tongue 175
33 Loosening of the Teeth 179
34 Blackening of the Teeth 185
35 Bruxism 189
36 Tooth Pain 197
37 Pain & Swelling of the Gums 207
38 Putrefying Gums 213
39 Atrophy of the Gums 219
40 Bleeding Gums 225

Bibliography, 231
Formula Index, 235
Symptom Index, 237

1
Bland Taste in the Mouth *(Kou Dan)*

Bland taste in the mouth is a subjective symptom in which the patient is unable to distinguish taste. It is very often accompanied by lack of pleasure in eating and reduced appetite. In most cases, the spleen and stomach are to blame for this complaint.

Disease causes, disease mechanisms:

"The stomach governs intake", while the spleen governs movement and transformation and opening into the portal of the mouth. "The spleen and stomach hold the office of the granaries from whence the five flavours emanate." Only if the spleen and stomach are harmonious is one able to taste food. If there is spleen-stomach disharmony, there will be a bland taste in the mouth.

I. Spleen-stomach vacuity

Spleen-stomach vacuity may be constitutional or caused by dietary irregularities which damage the spleen and stomach. It may also be due to enduring disease, in which case the spleen and stomach fail to be fortified. When the spleen and stomach are vacuous, spleen-stomach qi fails to go up to the mouth, and thus there is a bland taste in the mouth.

2. Dampness obstructing the middle burner

Dampness mainly comes from dietary irregularities which damage the spleen and stomach or from enduring exposure to dampness. If dampness obstructs in the middle burner, the spleen's movement and transformation will be impaired. As a result, dampness may be further engendered and accumulate. If dampness flows upward to the mouth, a bland taste in the mouth will occur.

3. Early stage damp warmth

When damp evils attack the body, they are likely to encumber the spleen. In the early stage of a damp warmth contraction, the spleen will be encumbered and the movement and transformation of the spleen will be damaged. This then leads to a failure in the transformation of dampness. If this damp warmth brews internally and affects the upbearing and downbearing of the qi mechanism, there will be a bland taste in the mouth.

Treatment based on pattern discrimination:

I. Spleen-stomach vacuity

Symptoms: A bland taste in the mouth, no pleasure in eating, and poor appetite accompanied by lack of strength and shortness of breath, exhaustion of the essence spirit, fullness and oppression in the stomach and abdomen, abdominal distention and loose stool, a pale, fat, tender tongue with thin fur, and a slow, weak pulse

Therapeutic principles: Fortify the spleen and boost the qi

Acupuncture & moxibustion:

Zhong Wan (CV 12)   Harmonizes the stomach qi

Zu San Li (St 36)   Together, these points fortify the spleen and
Gong Sun (Sp 4)   stomach and boost the qi.

Wei Shu (Bl 21)   Together, these points fortify the spleen and
Zhong Wan (CV 12)   stomach *Pi Shu* (Bl 20) and boost the qi. These
                             are used as alternatives to the above three points.
                             Use moxibustion, 7-10 cones each point.

Chinese medicinal formula: *Xiang Sha Liu Jun Zi Tang* (Aucklandia & Amomum Six Gentlemen Decoction)

2

Ingredients: Rice stir-fried Radix Codonopsitis Pilosulae (*Dang Shen*), 9g, bran stir-fried Rhizoma Atractylodis Macrocephalae (*Bai Zhu*), 9g, Sclerotium Poriae Cocos (*Fu Ling*), 6g, mix-fried Radix Glycyrrhizae (*Zhi Gan Cao*), 6g, stir-fried Pericarpium Citri Reticulatae (*Chen Pi*), 6g, lime-processed Rhizoma Pinelliae Ternatae (*Ban Xia*), 9g, uncooked Radix Auklandiae Lappae (*Mu Xiang*), 6g, Fructus Amomi (*Sha Ren*) 3g

Additions & subtractions: If the bland taste is severe, add Herba Agastachis Seu Pogostemi (*Huo Xiang*), 9g, and Herba Eupatorii Fortunei (*Pei Lan*), 9g. If poor appetite and loose stools are severe, add stir-fried Semen Nelumbinis Nuciferae (*Lian Zi*), 9g, and stir-fried Radix Dioscoreae Oppositae (*Shan Yao*), 9g. If there is chronic diarrhea, add stir-fried Radix Astragali Membranacei (*Huang Qi*), 12g, and mix-fried Rhizoma Cimicifugae (*Sheng Ma*), 3g.

2. Dampness obstructing the middle burner

Symptoms: A bland taste, stickiness, and sliminess in the mouth, reduced appetite, glomus and oppression in the chest and epigastrium, qi counterflow with nausea and vomiting, white or yellow, slimy tongue fur, and a soggy pulse

Therapeutic principles: Transform turbidity with aromatic (medicinals), arouse the spleen, and harmonize the center

Acupuncture & moxibustion:

Nei Guan (Per 6) *Zhong Wan* (CV 12)	Together, these points harmonize the center.
Zu San Li (St 36) *Yin Jiao* (Sp 6)	Together, these points arouse the spleen and *San* transform turbidity.

Chinese medicinal formula: Modified *Ping Wei San* (Level [*i.e.*, Calm] the Stomach Powder)

Ingredients: Herba Agastachis Seu Pogostemi (*Huo Xiang*), 9g, Herba Eupatorii Fortunei (*Pei Lan*), 9g, bran stir-fried Rhizoma Atractylodis (*Cang Zhu*), 12g, ginger mix-fried Cortex Magnoliae Officinalis (*Hou*

Po), 9g, stir-fried Pericarpium Citri Reticulatae (*Chen Pi*), 9g, uncooked Rhizoma Zingiberis (*Sheng Jiang*), 6g, Radix Glycyrrhizae (*Gan Cao*), 3g

Additions & subtractions: If there is damp heat, add Rhizoma Coptidis Chinensis (*Huang Lian*), 6g, and Radix Scutellariae Baicalensis (*Huang Qin*), 6g. If there is cold dampness, add dry Rhizoma Zingiberis (*Gan Jiang*), 6g, and Cortex Cinnamomi Cassiae (*Rou Gui*) 3g.

3. Early stage damp warmth

Symptoms: A bland taste, stickiness, and sliminess in the mouth, fever with aversion to cold, fatigue and lassitude, glomus and fullness in the chest and lateral costal regions, thin, white tongue fur, and a soggy, slow pulse

Acupuncture & moxibustion:

Kong Zui (Lu 6)
He Gu (LI 4)
Together, these points clear and transform the damp warmth and resolve the exterior.

Zhong Wan (CV 12)
Zu San Li (St 36)
Together, these points fortify the spleen and harmonize the stomach, transform dampness and downbear turbidity.

Zhi Gou (TB 6)
Frees the qi mechanism of the three burners to help clear and transform dampness and warmth

Additions & subtractions: For high fever, add *Da Zhui* (GV 14). For predominant dampness, add *Yin Ling Quan* (Sp 6). For fatigue and lassitude, add *Zu San Li* (St 36) and *Gao Huang* (Bl 43).

Chinese medicinal formula: Modified *Huo Po Xia Ling Tang* (Agastaches, Magnolia, Pinellia & Poria Decoction)

Ingredients: Herba Lophatheri Gracilis (*Dan Zhu Ye*), 12g, Herba Agastachis Seu Pogostemi (*Huo Xiang*), 6g, lime-processed Rhizoma Pinelliae Ternatae (*Ban Xia*), 6g, Sclerotium Poriae Cocos (*Fu Ling*), 9g, ginger mix-fried Cortex Magnoliae Officinalis (*Hou Po*), 6g, Semen Pruni Armeniacae (*Xing Ren*), 6g, uncooked Semen Coicis Lachryma-jobi (*Yi Yi Ren*), 15g, Fructus Cardamomi (*Bai Dou Kou*), 6g, Sclerotium Polypori Umbellati (*Zhu Ling*), 6g, Semen Praeparatus Sojae (*Dan Dou Chi*), 9g, Rhizoma Alismatis (*Ze Xie*), 6g

Remarks: Clinical practice shows that often these patterns are combined with food stagnating in the stomach duct. Hence, we should add Fructus Crataegi (*Shan Zha*) in case of meat, fish, or greasy food stagnation, Fructus Germinatus Hordei Vulgaris (*Mai Ya*) in case of vegetable, fruit, or cereal food stagnation, Semen Raphani Sativi (*Lai Fu Zi*) in case of food and qi stagnation, and Endothelium Corneum Gigeriae Galli (*Ji Nei Jin*) in case of food stagnation with qi vacuity.

Herba Eupatorii Fortunei (*Pei Lan*) and Herba Agastachis Seu Pogostemi (*Huo Xiang*) are really the best Chinese medicinals to treat a bland or sweet taste in the mouth and can be added to formulas for this condition. However, being aromatic, Eupatorium Agastaches should only be decocted briefly. The other main Chinese medicinals for this condition are Rhizoma Atractylodis (*Cang Zhu*), Rhizoma Atractylodis Macrocephalae (*Bai Zhu*), Semen Dolichoris Lablab (*Bai Bian Dou*), Sclerotium Poriae Cocos (*Fu Ling*), and Semen Coicis Lachryma-jobi (*Yi Yi Ren*).

If a bland taste is accompanied by excessive saliva caused by spleen-stomach vacuity cold, a remarkable Chinese medicine is Fructus Alpiniae Oxyphyllae (*Yi Zhi Ren*).

2
Bitter Taste in the Mouth (*Kou Ku*)

This is a subjective symptom where the patient has a bitter taste in their mouth even though no bitter foods or drinks have been taken in. This bitter taste in the mouth may be continuous, but frequently it is only noticeable on arising in the morning and before brushing the teeth.

Disease causes, disease mechanisms:

A bitter taste in the mouth is often caused by liver-gallbladder heat which forces the bile to flow upward.

1. Evils entering the *shao yang*

This pattern is often seen in cold damage disease when a *tai yang* pattern has failed to be resolved. Unresolved, the evils may pass to the *shao yang* which pertains to the gallbladder. If the evils transform into heat and steam the bile, the bile may counterflow upward to the mouth. Therefore, there is a bitter taste in the mouth.

2. Liver-gallbladder depressive heat

The liver governs coursing and discharge and likes orderly reaching. Emotional depression or enduring excesses of the five affects may transform into fire. When fire forces the bile to counterflow upward, a bitter taste in the mouth will occur.

Treatment based on pattern discrimination:

I. Evils entering the *shao yang*

Symptoms: A bitter taste in the mouth and dry throat, dizziness and vertigo, fullness in the chest and poor appetite, alternating fever and chills, thin, white tongue fur, and a wiry pulse

Therapeutic principles: Harmonize and resolve the *shao yang*

Acupuncture & moxibustion:

Yang Chi (TB 4) *Nei Guan* (Per 6)	Together, by combining the exterior and interior, these points free the flow of qi of the hand *shao yang* to harmonize and resolve the *shao yang* and thus harmonize stomach qi.
Qiu Xu (GB 40) *Li Gou* (Liv 5)	Together, by combining the exterior and interior, these points reinforce the action of harmonizing and resolving the *shao yang*.

Additions & subtractions: For headache, add *Feng Chi* (GB 20). For a persistent bitter taste in the mouth, add *Yang Ling Quan* (GB 34).

Note: Puncture the first two points before needling the last two.

Chinese medicinal formula: *Xiao Chai Hu Tang* (Minor Bupleurum Decoction)

Ingredients: Uncooked Radix Bupleuri (*Chai Hu*), 12g, uncooked Radix Scutellariae Baicalensis (*Huang Qin*), 9g, lime-processed Rhizoma Pinelliae Ternatae (*Ban Xia*), 9g, uncooked Radix Codonopsitis Pilosulae (*Dang Shen*), 6g, Radix Glycyrrhizae (*Gan Cao*), 3g, uncooked Rhizoma Zingiberis (*Sheng Jiang*), 9g, Fructus Zizyphi Jujubae (*Da Zao*), 4 pieces

2. Liver-gallbladder depressive heat

Symptoms: A bitter taste in the mouth, vexation and irascibility, headache and vertigo, red face and eyes, distention and fullness in the chest and

8

lateral costal regions; in some cases, genital swelling, pudendal itching, increased vaginal discharge, and/or turbid dribbling urination due to damp-heat pouring down; a red tongue with yellow fur and a wiry, rapid pulse

Therapeutic principles: Clear and drain the liver-gallbladder

Acupuncture & moxibustion:

Yang Ling Quan (GB 34)   An effective point for bitter taste in the mouth, clears heat in the gallbladder channel.

Qi Men (Liv 14)   Together, these points resolve depression.
Tai Chong (Liv 3)

Zhong Ting (CV 16)   Together, these points clear replete heat in the
Xia Xi (GB 43)   liver and gallbladder.

Additions & subtractions: For headache, add *Han Yan* (GB 4) and *Xuan Lu* (GB 5). For dizziness and vertigo, add *Bai Hui* (GV 20) and *Feng Chi* (GB 20).

Chinese medicinal formula: Modified *Long Dan Xie Gan Tang* (Gentiana Drain the Liver Decoction)

Ingredients: Radix Gentianae Scabrae (*Long Dan Cao*), 6g, uncooked Radix Scutellariae Baicalensis (*Huang Qin*), 9g, uncooked Fructus Gardeniae Jasminoidis (*Zhi Zi*), 9g, uncooked Rhizoma Alismatis (*Ze Xie*), 12g, Caulis Akebiae (*Mu Tong*), 6g, Semen Plantaginis (*Che Qian Zi*), 9g, uncooked Radix Angelicae Sinensis (*Dang Gui*), 6g, uncooked Radix Rehmanniae (*Sheng Di*), 9g, uncooked Radix Bupleuri (*Chai Hu*), 6g, Radix Glycyrrhizae (*Gan Cao*), 6g, Herba Artemisiae Capillaris (*Yin Chen Hao*), 9g

Remarks: Although *Long Dan Xie Gan Tang* is typically the textbook standard formula for the above pattern, it is frequently too cold for patients with liver-gallbladder depressive heat. This pattern tends to be a chronic, enduring one and most Western patients have an accompanying weak and/or damp spleen. Therefore, *Xiao Chai Hu Tang* described above or *Dan Zhi Xiao Yao San* (Moutan & Gardenia Rambling Powder) are more often the correct guiding formulas for long-term use.

Western patients rarely come in with bitter taste in their mouth as their main complaint. However, it is an extremely important symptom for determining if simple liver depression has transformed into depressive heat. Since the bitter taste typically disappears after the patient has brushed their teeth and eaten except for cases of real replete dampness and heat, such as in jaundice and cholecystitis, it is important to ask whether or not the patient experiences a bitter taste in their mouth on arising if depressive heat is suspected. Otherwise, by simply asking if there is a bitter taste in the mouth, the patient may give a false negative answer. A bitter taste in the mouth is the most commonly met of the abnormal tastes in the mouth in clinical practice.

The best Chinese medicinals for a bitter taste in the mouth are: Radix Scutellariae Baicalensis (*Huang Qin*) for gallbladder depressive heat, Radix Gentianae (*Long Dan Cao*) for liver-gallbladder fire and/or depressive heat, and Herba Artemisiae Capillaris (*Yin Chen Hao*) for damp heat. Two other good Chinese medicinals are Rhizoma Coptidis Chinensis (*Huang Lian*) and Fructus Gardeniae Jasminoidis (*Zhi Zi*).

3
Salty Taste in the Mouth (*Kou Xian*)

A salty taste in the mouth is a subjective symptom where the patient keeps having a salty taste in their mouth although they have not taken in anything salty. It is also possible that sometimes the patient spits up phlegm-drool which tastes salty.

Disease causes, disease mechanisms:

According to five phase theory, the salty flavor is ascribed to the kidneys and thus, in most cases, a salty taste in the mouth is impugned to upward counterflow of kidney humor.

I. Kidney vacuity

This vacuity may come from sexual taxation, enduring diseases which involve the kidneys, or aging. With kidney vacuity, true yin and yang may be rendered debilitated. In such cases, if true yin is damaged, vacuous yang will ascend and take the kidney humor upward to the mouth. Hence there will be a salty taste in the mouth. If true yang is damaged, the vacuous kidneys will fail to secure and astringe. This may lead to the kidney humor to flood or spill over upward. As a result, a salty taste in the mouth may occur.

2. Spleen dampness failing to be transformed

Dampness may be due to either external contraction from enduring exposure to damp evils or to spleen vacuity from dietary irregularities. The spleen governs water dampness, moistens the lower, and engenders the salty. If there is spleen dampness, the spleen can not transform water and, therefore, a salty taste in the mouth may occur.

Treatment based on pattern discrimination:

I. Kidney yin vacuity

Symptoms: A salty taste in the mouth or possibly sometimes spitting drool that tastes salty, dizziness, tinnitus, dry mouth and throat, pain and weakness of the low back and knees, vexatious heat in the five hearts, reduced sleep and profuse dreaming, a red tongue with reduced fur, and a fine, rapid pulse

Therapeutic principles: Enrich yin and downbear fire

Acupuncture & moxibustion:

Tai Xi (Ki 3) *Ran Gu* (Ki 2)	Together, these points enrich kidney yin and downbear fire to bring the kidney humor back to its source.
San Yin Jiao (Sp 6)	Enriches yin and downbears fire
Shen Shu (Bl 23) *Ming Men* (GV 4)	Together, these points supplement the kidney qi to gain yin from yang.

Chinese medicinal formula: Modified *Zhi Bai Di Huang Wan* (Anemarrhena & Phellodendron Rehmannia Pills)

Ingredients: Salt mix-fried Rhizoma Anemarrhenae Asphodeloidis (*Zhi Mu*), 9g, salt mix-fried Cortex Phellodendri (*Huang Bai*), 9g, prepared Radix Rehmanniae (*Shu Di*), 18g, steamed Fructus Corni Officinalis (*Shan Zhu Yu*), 12g, stir-fried Radix Dioscoreae Oppositae (*Shan Yao*), 12g, Sclerotium Poriae Cocos (*Fu Ling*), 9g, salt mix-fried Rhizoma Alismatis (*Ze Xie*), 9g, Cortex Radicis Moutan (*Dan Pi*), 9g, salt mix-fried Radix Achyranthis Bidentatae (*Niu Xi*), 9g

2. Kidney yang vacuity

Symptoms: A salty taste in the mouth, fatigue and lack of strength, shortage of qi with disinclination to speak, fear of cold, cold limbs, cold pain of the low back and knees, frequent urination at night, a pale, fat, tender tongue with teeth prints and white, watery, slimy fur, and a deep, fine, forceless pulse

Therapeutic principles: Warm and supplement kidney yang

Acupuncture & moxibustion:

Fu Liu (Ki 7)   Together, these points gain yang from yin.
Tai Xi (Ki 3)

Shen Shu (Bl 23)   Together, these points supplement kidney yang.
Ming Men (GV 4)   Use moxibustion on the head of the needles.
Qi Hai (CV 6)

Chinese medicinal formula: Modified *Shen Qi Wan* (Kidney Qi Pills)

Ingredients: Prepared Radix Rehmanniae (*Shu Di*), 18g, stir-fried Radix Dioscoreae Oppositae (*Shan Yao*), 12g, steamed Fructus Corni Officinalis (*Shan Zhu Yu*), 12g, salt mix-fried Rhizoma Alismatis (*Ze Xie*), 9g, Sclerotium Poriae Cocos (*Fu Ling*), 9g, Cortex Radicis Moutan (*Dan Pi*), 9g, Cortex Cinnamomi Cassiae (*Rou Gui*), 3g, bland Radix Lateralis Praeparatus Aconiti Carmichaeli (*Fu Zi*), 3g, uncooked Fructus Schisandrae Chinensis (*Wu Wei Zi*), 6g

3. Spleen dampness failing to be transformed

Symptoms: A salty taste associated with stickiness and sliminess in the mouth, no desire for drinking water, torpid intake, a bag-over-the-head sensation or the feeling of a tight band around the head, cumbersome limbs, short voidings of scant urine, a pale tongue with white, slimy fur, and a slippery pulse

Therapeutic principles: Arouse the spleen and transform dampness

Acupuncture & moxibustion:

Shui Fen (CV 9)   Together, these points disinhibit dampness.
Yin Ling Quan (Sp 9)
San Yin Jiao (Sp 6)

Zhong Wan (CV 12)	Together, these points arouse the spleen and
Zu San Li (St 36)	transform dampness.

Chinese medicinal formula: Modified *Er Chen Tang* (Two Aged [Ingredients] Decoction)

Ingredients: Lime-processed Rhizoma Pinelliae Ternatae (*Ban Xia*), 9g, Pericarpium Citri Reticulatae (*Chen Pi*), 9g, Sclerotium Poriae Cocos (*Fu Ling*) 9g, mix-fried Radix Glycyrrhizae (*Zhi Gan Cao*), 3g, Herba Agastachis Seu Pogostemi (*Huo Xiang*), 9g, Sclerotium Polypori Umbellati (*Zhu Ling*), 6g, Lignum Santali Albi (*Tan Xiang*), 3g, processed Fructus Evodiae Rutecarpae (*Wu Zhu Yu*), 3g

4
Sour Taste in the Mouth (*Kou Suan*)

A sour taste in the mouth is a subjective symptom. It refers to a sour taste in the mouth even though nothing sour has been taken in. In some severe cases, there is also sour smell which can be sensed in the mouth.

Disease causes, disease mechanisms:

I. Liver heat

Liver heat mainly comes from emotional disturbance which transforms fire or engenders heat. The sour flavor is associated with the liver. If liver heat brews internally and steams upward, a sour taste may occur in the mouth.

2. Spleen vacuity being exploited by wood

According to five phase theory, the liver checks the spleen. If the spleen is vacuous, the liver may overwhelm the spleen. Usually a bland or sweet taste is associated with spleen vacuity. However, if there is liver exuberance, the sour taste may become predominant since the sour taste is associated with the liver. Therefore, a sour taste may occur in the mouth when an exuberant liver overwhelms a vacuous spleen.

3. Food stagnating in the stomach duct

Over-intake of food or intake of unclean food may cause food stagnating in the stomach duct and damage the spleen and stomach. This may then lead to failure of the spleen's movement and transformation. Consequently, the water and grain taken in cannot be moved and transformed properly. Hence, there may be a sour taste in the mouth.

Treatment based on pattern discrimination:

I. Liver heat

Symptoms: Sour and bitter tastes in the mouth, vertigo, tinnitus, red face and eyes, vexation and agitation, irascibility, pain and fullness in the chest and lateral costal regions, dry stool, yellow urine (*i.e.,* darker than normal colored urine), thin, yellow tongue fur, and a wiry, rapid pulse

Therapeutic principles: Course the liver and clear heat

Acupuncture & moxibustion:

Yang Ling Quan (GB 34) *Yang Fu* (GB 38)	An effective point for sour and bitter tastes in the mouth; together with *Yang Fu*, clears the liver and disinhibits the gallbladder.
Qi Men (Liv 14) *Tai Chong* (Liv 3)	Together, these points course the liver and resolve depression.
Xia Xi (GB 43)	Clears replete heat in the liver-gallbladder

Chinese medicinal formula: Modified *Chai Hu Qing Gan Yin* (Bupleurum Clear Liver Drink)

Ingredients: Uncooked Radix Bupleuri (*Chai Hu*), 9g, uncooked Radix Scutellariae Baicalensis (*Huang Qin*), 9g, uncooked Fructus Gardeniae Jasminoidis (*Zhi Zi*), 9g, uncooked Rhizoma Coptidis Chinensis (*Huang Lian*), 6g, processed Fructus Evodiae Rutecarpae (*Wu Zhu Yu*), 3g, uncooked Radix Rehmanniae (*Sheng Di*), 9g, Cortex Radicis Moutan (*Dan Pi*), 6g, uncooked Radix Albus Paeoniae Lactiflorae (*Bai Shao*), 6g, Radix Glycyrrhizae (*Gan Cao*), 6g

Additions & subtractions: If there is acid regurgitation or a severe sour taste in the mouth, add Os Sepiae Seu Sepiellae (*Hai Piao Xiao*), 9g, and Bulbus Fritillariae Thunbergii (*Zhe Bei Mu*), 9g. If there is severe constipation, add Herba Aloes (*Lu Hui*), 1g, powdered.

2. Spleen vacuity being exploited by wood

Symptoms: A sour taste in the mouth or sometimes sour belching, poor appetite, abdominal distention, loose stools, fatigue and lack of strength, pain and distention in the lateral costal regions, frequent sighing, white tongue fur, and a wiry, fine pulse

Therapeutic principles: Fortify the spleen and regulate the liver

Acupuncture & moxibustion:

Ri Yue (GB 24) *Qi Men* (Liv 14)	Together, these points course and regulate the liver. *Ri Yue* is an effective point for sour taste in the mouth.
Pi Shu (Bl 20) *Wei Shu* (Bl 21) *Gong Sun* (Sp 4)	Together, these points fortify the spleen.

Additions and subtractions: For fatigue and lack of strength, add *Zu San Li* (St 36).

Chinese medicinal formula: *Liu Jun Zi Tang* (Six Gentlemen Decoction) plus *Zuo Jin Wan* (Left Metal Pills)

Ingredients: Honey stir-fried Radix Codonopsitis Pilosulae (*Dang Shen*), 9g, bran stir-fried Rhizoma Atractylodis Macrocephalae (*Bai Zhu*), 9g, Sclerotium Poriae Cocos (*Fu Ling*), 9g, mix-fried Radix Glycyrrhizae (*Zhi Gan Cao*), 6g, lime-processed Rhizoma Pinelliae Ternatae (*Ban Xia*), 9g, stir-fried Pericarpium Citri Reticulatae (*Chen Pi*), 9g, uncooked Rhizoma Coptidis Chinensis (*Huang Lian*), 6g, processed Fructus Evodiae Rutecarpae (*Wu Zhu Yu*), 2g

3. Food stagnating in the stomach duct

Symptoms: A sour taste in the mouth sometimes with putrid belching, distention and oppression in the stomach and abdomen, no thought of food or drink, constipation or diarrhea with putrid-smelling stools, yellow, slimy tongue fur, and a slippery pulse

Therapeutic principles: Disperse food and abduct stagnation

Acupuncture & moxibustion:

Zu San Li (St 36)	An effective point for sour taste in the mouth due
Xia Wan (CV 10)	to food stagnation; together with *Xia Wan* and
Liang Men (St 21)	*Liang Men*, disperses food.

Tian Shu (St 25)	Together, these points rectify the qi, abduct
Nei Ting (St 44)	stagnation, and clear heat from food stagnation to help sour taste.

Additions & subtractions: For meat stagnation, use *Hua Rou Men* (St 24) instead of *Liang Men*.

Chinese medicinal formula: Modified *Bao He Wan* (Preserve Harmony Pills)

Ingredients: Stir-fried Fructus Crataegi (*Shan Zha*), 18g, stir-fried Massa Medica Fermentata (*Shen Qu*), 6g, lime-processed Rhizoma Pinelliae Ternatae (*Ban Xia*), 9g, stir-fried Pericarpium Citri Reticulatae (*Chen Pi*), 9g, Sclerotium Poriae Cocos (*Fu Ling*), 9g, Fructus Forsythiae Suspensae (*Lian Qiao*), 9g, Semen Raphani Sativi (*Lai Fu Zi*) 9g, Fructus Citri Aurantii (*Zhi Ke*), 6g

Additions & subtractions: For spleen vacuity, add bran stir-fried Rhizoma Atractylodis Macrocephalae (*Bai Zhu*), 9g. For constipation, add uncooked Radix Et Rhizoma Rhei (*Da Huang*), 6-9g. If there is acid regurgitation or a severe sour taste in the mouth, add Os Sepiae Seu Sepiellae (*Hai Piao Xiao*), 9g, and Bulbus Fritillariae Thunbergii (*Zhe Bei Mu*), 9g.

Remarks: Similar to a bland taste in the mouth, many cases of a sour taste in the mouth are accompanied by food stagnation. Therefore, the same Chinese medicinals are often added for the various types of food stagnation. Two combinations of Chinese medicinals are especially effective for a sour taste in the mouth:

a. Rhizoma Coptidis Chinensis (*Huang Lian*), 6g, and Fructus Evodiae Rutecarpae (*Wu Zhu Yu*), 2g. This combination forms *Zuo Jin Wang* (Left Metal Pills). This is a very effective combination and can be prescribed in any case: vacuity or repletion, heat or cold. However, if heat predominates, use a larger dosage of Coptis (*i.e.*, 7-9g). If cold predominates, use a larger dosage of Evodia, *(i.e.*, 3-5g). In case of stomach yin vacuity, add Herba Dendrobii (*Shi Hu*), 10g. In case of stomach qi vacuity, add Radix Codonopsitis Pilosulae (*Dang Shen*), 10g.

b. Os Sepiae Seu Sepiellae (*Hai Piao Xiao*), 10g in decoction or 3g in powder and Bulbus Fritillariae Thunbergii (*Zhe Bei Mu*), 10g in decoction or 3g in powder, is another effective combination for a sour taste in the mouth if it is accompanied by acid regurgitation and burning in the stomach. They have a pronounced antacid effect.

Other good Chinese antacid medicinals are Concha Arcae (*Wa Leng Zi*), Concha Meretricis Sinensis (*Hai Ge Ke*), and Concha Ostreae (*Mu Li*).

5
Burning or Peppery Taste in the Mouth (*Kou La*)

A burning or peppery taste in the mouth is a subjective symptom where the patient feels tingling and a pungent taste in the mouth.

Disease causes, disease mechanisms:

Lung heat fuming & steaming

This heat is mainly derived from externally contracted evils that enter the interior and then transform into heat. If the heat remains uncleared and brews in the lungs, it will fume and steam over time. Pepper is an acrid flavor and the acrid flavor is associated with the lungs. Thus, when lung heat fumes and steams, an acrid taste may occur in the mouth.

Treatment based on pattern discrimination:

Lung heat fuming & steaming

Symptoms: A burning or peppery, acrid taste in the mouth, often accompanied by a tingling sensation on the surface of the tongue, cough, rapid breathing, the breath sometimes smelling fishy, thirst, yellow urine, a red tongue with yellow fur, and a rapid pulse

Therapeutic principles: Clear and drain lung heat

Acupuncture & moxibustion:

Yu Ji (Lu 10)　　　　　Together, these points clear and drain lung heat.
Chi Ze (Lu 5)
Fei Shu (Bl 13)
Ge Shu (Bl 17)

He Gu (LI 4) *Qu Chi* (LI 11) — Together, these points help clear and drain lung heat.

Additions & subtractions: For cough, add *Zhong Fu* (Lu 1). For fever, add *Da Zhui* (GV 14).

Chinese medicinal formula: Modified *Xie Bai San* (Drain White Powder)

Ingredients: Cortex Radicis Mori Albi (*Sang Bai Pi*), 9g, Cortex Radicis Lycii Chinensis (*Di Gu Pi*), 9g, Radix Glycyrrhizae (*Gan Cao*) 9g, uncooked Radix Platycodi Grandiflori (*Jie Geng*), 9g, uncooked Rhizoma Anemarrhenae Asphodeloidis (*Zhi Mu*) 9g, uncooked Radix Scutellariae Baicalensis (*Huang Qin*), 6g, Tuber Ophiopogonis Japonici (*Mai Men Dong*), 6g

Additions & subtractions: For cough, add uncooked Fructus Schisandrae Chinensis (*Wu Wei Zi*), 12g.

Remarks: A burning or peppery, acrid taste in the mouth is not so uncommon a symptom. It is never a main complaint, but in clinical practice, it is common with wind heat or heat attacking the lung, especially when there is nasal inflammation or cough. In these cases, the sensation is located on the tip of the tongue in the area corresponding to the lungs.

6
Sweet Taste in the Mouth (*Kou Tian*)

This is a subjective symptom where the patient feels a sweet taste like sugar or honey in their mouth even though they have not ingested anything sweet.

Disease causes, disease mechanisms:

1. Spleen-stomach heat steaming

"Fatty food produces internal heat, while sweet food produces fullness in the center." Addiction to fatty and sweet food may engender internal heat. If this heat brews and binds in the spleen and stomach, contends with the grain qi, and steams upward, there will be a sweet taste in the mouth. In addition, externally contracted damp heat accumulating and brewing in the spleen and stomach can also contribute to this problem.

2. Spleen-stomach qi & yin dual vacuity

Aging and enduring diseases may lead to a dual vacuity of qi and yin. If these involve the spleen and stomach, there will be a dual vacuity of spleen-stomach qi and yin. Yin is responsible for checking yang. Therefore, if there is yin vacuity, internal heat is engendered. Spleen qi is responsible for moving and transforming the water and grain taken in. Thus, if there is spleen qi vacuity, water and grain will accumulate and engender dampness. If this internal heat binds with this dampness and then brews and steams upward, a sweet taste may occur in the mouth.[1]

---

[1] This pattern and complaint is frequent in some diabetics.

Treatment based on pattern discrimination:

I. Spleen-stomach heat steaming

Symptoms: A sweet taste in the mouth, dry mouth with desire to drink, large food intake with rapid hungering, dry stool, possible yellow urine in some cases, sores on the tongue and lips, a red tongue with yellow, dry fur, and a rapid, forceful pulse

Therapeutic principles: Clear and drain stomach heat

Acupuncture & moxibustion:

Li Dui (St 45) *Da Du* (Sp 2) *Nei Ting* (St 44) *Jie Xi* (St 41)	Together, these points clear and drain stomach heat by "withdrawing the fire wood from unde the pot."
San Yin Jiao (Sp 6) *Tai Xi* (Ki 3)	Together, these points supplement yin fluids to quench the fire.

Additions & subtractions: For constipation, add *Shang Ju Xu* (St 37). For red, swollen, painful tongue and lips, add *Lao Gong* (Per 8).

Chinese medicinal formula: Modified *Xie Huang San* (Drain the Yellow Powder)

Ingredients: Folium Agastachis Seu Pogostemi (*Huo Xiang Ye*)[2], 12g, Herba Eupatorii Fortunei (*Pei Lan*), 9g, Sclerotium Poriae Cocos (*Fu Ling*), 9g, uncooked Gypsum Fibrosum (*Shi Gao*), 15g, Radix Glycyrrhizae (*Gan Cao*), 6g, Radix Ledebouriellae Divaricatae (*Fang Feng*), 9g, uncooked Fructus Gardeniae Jasminoidis (*Zhi Zi*), 9g

---

[2] Folium Agastachis Seu Pogostemi (*Huo Xiang Ye*) is superior to Herba Agastachis Seu Pogostemi (*Huo Xiang*) for the treatment of sweet taste in the mouth. However, if one does not have Folium Agastachis, Herba Agastachis can be used with success.

Additions & subtractions: For severe spleen-stomach heat with red, cracked, painful mouth and tongue, add uncooked Rhizoma Coptidis Chinensis (*Huang Lian*), 6g, and uncooked Cortex Phellodendri (*Huang Bai*), 9g. If there is constipation, add uncooked Radix Et Rhizoma Rhei (*Da Huang*), 6g, and Mirabilitum (*Mang Xiao*), 6g.

2. Spleen-stomach qi & yin dual vacuity

Symptoms: A sweet taste in the mouth, no thought of food, a dry mouth with no desire to drink or, if there is any desire to drink, it is only for a little drink, lassitude of the spirit and lack of strength, distention in the stomach and abdomen, a red tongue with reduced fur, and a fine, rapid pulse

Therapeutic principles: Boost the qi and fortify the spleen, harmonize the stomach and nourish yin

Acupuncture & moxibustion:

Qi Hai (CV 6)	Together, these points boost the qi.
Guan Yuan (CV 4)	

Zu San Li (St 36)	Together, these points fortify the spleen and
Zhong Wan (CV 12)	harmonize the stomach. Together, these
San Yin Jiao (Sp 6)	points nourish yin.

Use alternatively with the following group:

Pi Shu (Bl 20)	Together, these points fortify the spleen and
Wei Shu (Bl 21)	stomach (qi and yin).

Qi Hai Shu (Bl 24)	Together, these points boost the qi.
Guan Yuan Shu (Bl 26)	

Chinese medicinal formula: Modified *Qi Wei Bai Zhu San* (Seven Flavors Atractylodes Powder)

Ingredients: Uncooked Radix Codonopsitis Pilosulae (*Dang Shen*), 9g, Sclerotium Poriae Cocos (*Fu Ling*), 9g, bran stir-fried Rhizoma Atractylodis Macrocephalae (*Bai Zhu*), 9g, mix-fried Radix Glycyrrhizae (*Zhi Gan Cao*), 6g, Herba Agastachis Seu Pogostemi (*Huo Xiang*), 6g, Herba Eupatorii Fortunei (*Pei Lan*), 6g, uncooked Radix Auklandiae Lappae (*Mu Xiang*), 6g, uncooked Radix Dioscoreae Oppositae (*Shan Yao*), 9g, Herba Dendrobii (*Shi Hu*), 9g, Semen Nelumbinis Nuciferae (*Lian Zi*), 9g

Remarks: Eupatorium, Herba Agastachis, and Folium Agastachis are the best Chinese medicinals for treating a sweet taste in the mouth. Eupatorium is the best of these, expecially for spleen-stomach heat steaming. This is also called spleen pure heat. Spleen pure heat is the steaming of harassing qi toward the mouth. It is caused by spleen heat generated by fatty and sweet foods.

One should keep in mind that to be efficient, these medicinals should only be decocted for a short time.

According to clinical experience, Radix Puerariae (*Ge Gen*) is another good Chinese medicinal for a sweet taste in the mouth.

7
Sliminess in the Mouth (*Kou Ni*)

Sliminess in the mouth is a subjective symptom where the patient feels stickiness and greasiness as if there were some tasteless, thin cream cheese in the mouth.

Disease causes, disease mechanisms:

The spleen is often to blame for sliminess in the mouth. The spleen governs the movement and transformation of water dampness. If one is addicted to raw, chilled, fatty, or sweat food or cold drinks or if there is enduring exposure to cold and dampness, the spleen-stomach may be damaged. This then leads to the spleen's failure to move and transform. As a result, damp turbidity will be engendered and accumulate. The spleen opens into the portal of the mouth. If damp turbidity spills over upwards, there will be sliminess in the mouth. If the damp turbidity accumulates in the middle burner, it may transform into damp heat over time. In that case, the sliminess in the mouth will be complicated by heat signs, while if the heat burns dampness into phlegm, there will also be symptoms of phlegm heat in addition to sliminess in the mouth.

Treatment based on pattern discrimination:

I. Cold dampness encumbering the spleen

Symptoms: A slimy and bland taste in the mouth, no thought of food or drink, fullness and oppression in the stomach and abdomen, fatigue and lack of strength, loose stools, scant urine, a pale tongue with white, slimy fur[3], and a slippery, soggy pulse

---

[3] In clinical practice, one frequently sees clear, grey fur.

Therapeutic principles: Fortify the spleen and dry dampness; transform turbidity with aromatic (medicinals)

Acupuncture & moxibustion:

Zhong Wan (CV 12)	Together, these points warm and dissipate cold.
Shen Que (CV 8)	Use moxibustion on the head of the needles.
Zu San Li (St 36)	Together, these points fortify the spleen and dry
Yin Ling Quan (Sp 6)	dampness.
Qi Hai (CV 6)	With moxibustion, boosts the qi to distribute fluids so as to transform dampness

Chinese medicinal formula: Modified *Ping Wei San* (Level [*i.e.*, Calm] the Stomach Powder)

Ingredients: Herba Agastachis Seu Pogostemi (*Huo Xiang*), 9g, Herba Eupatorii Fortunei (*Pei Lan*), 9g, Fructus Amomi (*Sha Ren*), 9g, Radix Auklandiae Lappae (*Mu Xiang*), 9g, bran stir-fried Rhizoma Atractylodis (*Cang Zhu*), 15g, ginger mix-fried Cortex Magnoliae Officinalis (*Hou Po*), 9g, stir-fried Pericarpium Citri Reticulatae (*Chen Pi*), 9g, uncooked Rhizoma Zingiberis (*Sheng Jiang*), 6g, Radix Glycyrrhizae (*Gan Cao*), 3g

2. Damp heat obstructing the center

Symptoms: Sliminess in the mouth with foul smell, thirst but no desire to drink, poor appetite, distention and fullness in the stomach and abdomen, reddish urine, loose stools, a red tongue with yellow, slimy fur, and a slippery, rapid pulse

Therapeutic principles: Clear heat, transform dampness, and arouse the spleen

Acupuncture & moxibustion:

Gong Sun (Sp 4)	Together, these points loosen the center and
Nei Guan (Per 6)	downbear turbidity.

Yin Ling Quan (Sp 9)	Together, these points arouse the spleen, clear
Zu San Li (St 36)	heat, and transform dampness.

Additions & subtractions: For bad breath, add *Da Ling* (Per 7).

Chinese medicinal formula: *Gan Lu Xiao Du Dan* (Sweet Dew Disperse Toxins Elixir)

Ingredients: Talcum (*Hua Shi*), 20g, Herba Artemisiae Capillaris (*Yin Chen Hao*), 12g, uncooked Radix Scutellariae Baicalensis (*Huang Qin*), 9g, Rhizoma Acori Graminei (*Shi Chang Pu*), 9g, Bulbus Fritillariae Cirrhosae (*Chuan Bei Mu*), 6g, Caulis Akebiae (*Mu Tong*), 5g, Herba Agastachis Seu Pogostemi (*Huo Xiang*), 9g, Rhizoma Belamcandae Chinensis (*She Gan*), 6g, Fructus Forsythiae Suspensae (*Lian Qiao*), 6g, Herba Menthae Haplocalysis (*Bo He*), 3g, Fructus Cardamomi (*Bai Dou Kou*), 6g

Additions & subtractions: If there is a bitter taste in the mouth, add Radix Gentianae Scabrae (*Long Dan Cao*), 6g, and Herba Artemisiae Capillaris (*Yin Chen Hao*), 9g.

3. Phlegm heat binding in the interior

Symptoms: Sliminess in the mouth, thirst with no desire to drink, fullness and oppression in the chest and diaphragm, vexation and disquietude, cough with thick, yellow phlegm which is difficult to expectorate, reduced food intake, torpid intake, short voidings of reddish urine, a red tongue with yellow, slimy fur, and a slippery, rapid pulse

Therapeutic principles: Clear heat and transform phlegm

Acupuncture & moxibustion:

Zhong Wan (CV 12) Together, these points loosen the center and
Jian Li (CV 11) transform turbidity.

Yin Ling Quan (Sp 9) Together, these points move the qi and transform
Shan Zhong (CV 17) dampness.

Feng Long (St 40) Together, these points clear heat and transform
Nei Ting (St 44) phlegm.

Additions & subtractions: For vexation and insomnia, add *Shen Men* (Ht 7) and *Nei Guan* (Per 6).

Chinese medicinal formula: *Qing Qi Hua Tan Wan* (Clear the Qi & Transform Phlegm Pills)

Ingredients: Fructus Trichosanthis Kirlowii (*Gua Lou*), 9g, uncooked Pericarpium Citri Reticulatae (*Chen Pi*), 9g, uncooked Radix Scutellariae Baicalensis (*Huang Qin*), 9g, Semen Pruni Armeniacae (*Xing Ren*), 9g, uncooked Fructus Immaturus Citri Aurantii (*Zhi Shi*), 9g, Sclerotium Poriae Cocos (*Fu Ling*), 9g, bile-processed Rhizoma Arisaematis (*Dan Nan Xing*), 12g, lime-processed Rhizoma Pinelliae Ternatae (*Ban Xia*), 12g

Remarks: Fructus Cardmomi (*Bai Dou Kou*) and Fructus Amomi (*Sha Ren*) are the best Chinese medicinals for sliminess in the mouth and especially for cold dampness encumbering the spleen. However, they can be used in the two other patterns in order to reinforce their formulas' effects. In this case, one should use the powdered form and add this to the decoction before drinking. This insures that the aromatic substances of these medicinals are not lost during decoction.

8
Malodorous Mouth (*Kou Chou*)

Malodorous mouth or bad breath refers to a foul smell to the breath.[4]

Disease causes, disease mechanisms:

I. Food stagnating in the stomach duct

Dietary irregularities and addiction to fatty and/or sweet food may damage the stomach and impair the movement of the stomach and intestines, resulting in food stagnation in the stomach duct. "The stomach governs intake and rottening and ripening" and stomach qi should descend. When damaged, the stomach can not rotten or ripen and send down the food taken in properly. Therefore, the stagnated food turns foul. Since it cannot descend, the stomach qi must go upward, giving rise to halitosis.

2. Stomach fire steaming upward

Addiction to acrid food and/or food with rich flavor or external contraction of warm heat evils which enter the *yang ming* may result in stomach fire. If fire brews in the stomach and becomes exuberant, it will steam upward to burn the gums and putrefy the blood there, thus leading to halitosis.

3. Phlegm heat congesting in the lungs

Phlegm heat may be due to externally contracted evils which enter the interior, transform into fire, and burn the fluids into phlegm or to phlegm accumulating in the lungs transforming heat over time. If phlegm heat

---

[4] If bad breath has a specific bad odor, for instance a sour odor, it is better to approach the complaint from the point of view of a sour taste in the mouth.

congesting in the lungs endures, it may burn and damage the qi and blood of the lungs, thus giving rise to *yong* of the lungs. Halitosis occurs when fire putrefies the blood into pus.

4. Liver-stomach disharmony

Due to emotional stress and frustration, liver depression may transform into depressive heat. This may then cause stomach depressive heat which results in bad breath.

Treatment based on pattern discrimination:

I. Food stagnating in the stomach duct

Symptoms: Bad breath with sour smell, putrid belching and acid regurgitation, distention and fullness and/or pain in the stomach and abdomen, constipation or diarrhea with untransformed food in the stools, flatulence with foul smell, thick, slimy tongue fur, and a slippery pulse

Therapeutic principles: Disperse food and abduct stagnation

Acupuncture & moxibustion:

Xia Wan (CV 10) *Liang Men* (St 21)	Together, these points disperse food, free the flow, and downbear stomach qi.
Tian Shu (St 25) *Shang Ju Xu* (St 37)	Together, these points free the bowels and abduct stagnation.
Zhi Gou (TB 6)	Moves the qi and abducts stagnation

Chinese medicinal formula: Modified *Bao He Wan* (Preserve Harmony Pills)

Ingredients: Stir-fried Fructus Crataegi (*Shan Zha*), 9g, stir-fried Massa Medica Fermentata (*Shen Qu*), 9g, lime-processed Rhizoma Pinelliae Ternatae (*Ban Xia*), 9g, stir-fried Pericarpium Citri Reticulatae (*Chen Pi*), 6g, Sclerotium Poriae Cocos (*Fu Ling*), 9g, Fructus Forsythiae Suspensae

(*Lian Qiao*), 9g, Semen Raphani Sativi (*Lai Fu Zi*) 9g, stir-fried till scorched Semen Arecae Catechu (*Bing Lang*), 9g, Fructus Cardamomi (*Cao Dou Kou*), 6g[5]

2. Stomach fire steaming upward

Symptoms: Bad breath, thirst with liking for chilled drinks, painful, swollen gums or putrid gums with discharge of pus and blood, constipation, yellow urine, a red tongue with yellow fur, and a rapid, forceful pulse

Therapeutic principles: Clear and discharge stomach fire

Acupuncture & moxibustion:

Lian Quan (CV 23)   Together, these points clear heat and drain fire.
Ren Zhong (GV 26)

Da Ling (Per 7)   Together, these points clear and downbear
Feng Long (St 40)   stomach fire.
Nei Ting (St 44)

Additions & subtractions: For constipation, add *Tian Shu* (St 25). For toothache, add *Da Ying* (St 5).

Chinese medicinal formula: Modified *Qing Wei San* (Clear the Stomach Powder)

Ingredients: Uncooked Gypsum Fibrosum (*Shi Gao*), 20g, uncooked Radix Scutellariae Baicalensis (*Huang Qin*), 9g, uncooked Rhizoma Coptidis Chinensis (*Huang Lian*), 6g, uncooked Radix Rehmanniae (*Sheng Di*), 9g, Cortex Radicis Moutan (*Dan Pi*), 9g, uncooked Rhizoma Cimicifugae (*Sheng Ma*), 6g

---

[5] Cardomon is an effective Chinese medicinal for treating malodorous mouth, but it is especially useful for bad breath coming from the digestive tract. A simple and popular formula is Fructus Cardamomi (*Cao Dou Kou*) 3g and Herba Asari Cum Radice (*Xi Xin*) 1g, both powdered. Take this 3 times each day, after meals.

3. Phlegm heat congesting in the lungs

Symptoms: Bad breath with a fishy smell, pain and distention in the chest, cough with expectoration of fishy smelling, turbid phlegm or pus and blood, dry mouth with no desire to drink, yellow, slimy tongue fur, and a slippery, rapid pulse

Therapeutic principles: Clear the lungs and transform phlegm

Acupuncture & moxibustion:

Lie Que (Lu 7) *Yu Ji* (Lu 10) *Tong Li* (Ht 5)	Together, these points clear heat in the upper burner, especially in the lungs.
Zhi Gou (TB 6) *Feng Long* (St 40)	Together, these points move the qi and transform phlegm.

Additions & subtractions: For fever, add *Zhong Fu* (Lu 1) and *Fei Shu* (Bl 13).

Note: For lung *yong* (*i.e.*, pulmonary abscess), acupuncture is only a complement to internally administered Chinese medicinal formulas.

Chinese medicinal formula: Modified *Wei Jing Tang* (Phragmites Decoction)

Ingredients: Rhizoma Phragmitis Communis (*Lu Gen*), 30g, uncooked Semen Coicis Lachryma-jobi (*Yi Yi Ren*), 20g, Semen Benincasae Hispidae (*Dong Gua Zi*), 15g, scalded Semen Pruni Persicae (*Tao Ren*), 9g, Bulbus Fritillariae Cirrhosae (*Chuan Bei Mu*), 9g, uncooked Radix Platycodi Grandiflori (*Jie Geng*), 9g, Flos Lonicerae Japonicae (*Jin Yin Hua*), 9g, Herba Houttuyniae Cordatae Cum Radice (*Yu Xing Cao*), 15g, Radix Glycyrrhizae (*Gan Cao*), 6g

4. Liver-stomach disharmony

Symptoms: Bad breath, belching and burping, possible acid regurgitation, chest oppression and lateral costal distention and pain, worse with stress, irritability, a normal tongue with thin, white or slightly yellow fur, and a bowstring, wiry pulse

Therapeutic principles: Course the liver and rectify the qi, clear heat and harmonize the stomach

Acupuncture & moxibustion:

Tai Chong (Liv 3) *He Gu* (LI 4)	Together, these points course the liver and rectify the qi.
Nei Ting (St 44) *Zu San Li* (St 36)	Together, these points clear heat and harmonize the stomach.
Zhong Wan (CV 12)	Harmonizes the stomach
Zhang Men (Liv 13)	Courses the liver and disperses distention

Chinese medicinal formula: Modified *Chai Hu Shu Gan San* (Bupleurum Sooth the Liver Powder)

Ingredients: Radix Bupleuri (*Chai Hu*), 9-12g, Radix Albus Paeoniae Lactiflorae (*Bai Shao*), 6-9g, Fructus Citri Aurantii (*Zhi Ke*), 6-9g, Radix Ligusticum Wallichii (*Chuan Xiong*), 3-6g, Rhizoma Cyperi Rotundi (*Xiang Fu*), 6-9g, Radix Scutellariae Baicalensis (*Huang Qin*), 9-12g, Radix Glycyrrhizae (*Gan Cao*), 1-3g

Additions: If heat is more severe, add Rhizoma Coptidis Chinensis (*Huang Lian*), 3g. If abdominal pain is more severe, add Rhizoma Corydalis Yanhusuo (*Yan Hu Suo*), 15g. If there is belching and acid regurgitation, add Concha Arcae (*Wa Leng Zi*) and Os Sepiae Seu Sepiellae (*Wu Zei Gu*).

9
Oral Thirst (*Kou Ke*)

Oral thirst refers to the subjective feeling of dryness in the mouth accompanied, in most cases, by a desire or need to drink. In some cases, the patient may complain of dryness in the mouth with no desire to drink. This is called "pseudo-thirst."

Disease causes, disease mechanisms:

Thirst is a very commonly encountered symptom in clinical practice. It may be due to either external or internal causes. Though the disease cause is often heat evils which burn and damage liquids, it is not rare that qi vacuity and water retention contribute to this problem. Although its disease causes can be many, all these result in one basic disease mechanism: lack of liquid in the mouth.

1. Contraction of external evils

Externally contracted heat evils or any other external evils that transform into heat after entering the body may damage liquids, leading to a lack of liquids in general (*i.e.*, in the whole body). If there is a general lack of liquids, the mouth will not be nourished sufficiently and thus there will be thirst with desire to drink.

2. Internal heat or fire

Addiction to acrid food, enduring exposure to sunlight in summer, or hot working conditions may result in replete heat, while aging or enduring disease may render yin vacuous, leading to vacuity heat. Heat, whether replete or vacuous, is a yang evil which eventually damages yin liquids. When liquids are damaged, there will be thirst.

3. Liquids failing to ascend & moisten the mouth

Water rheum collecting internally or blood stasis in the interior can prevent liquids from ascending to nourish the mouth by blocking and obstructing the channels, while qi vacuity unable to upbear can also result in failure to distribute liquids above. If liquids cannot ascend and moisten the mouth due to water rheum collecting and blood stasis in the interior, there will be thirst. But the thirst will not be accompanied by a desire to drink unless water rheum collection and blood stasis are accompanied by heat. In that case, there may be desire for scanty drink. If thirst is due to vacuous qi failing to distribute liquids to the mouth, this thirst is often accompanied by a desire to drink but a desire to drink warm drinks. This is because qi is yang in nature and if there is a qi vacuity, there is lack of righteous heat.

4. Damp heat fuming & steaming

Addiction to fatty and/or sweet food or contraction of external damp heat may result in damp heat fuming and steaming. Both dampness and heat can set in motion mechanisms resulting in oral thirst. If dampness encumbers the spleen, the spleen cannot transform water and grain. In that case, liquids will be hindered from being moved upward to the mouth since dampness and untransformed water may block the channels. The yang heat of damp heat may directly damage yin liquids. In addition, the combination of dampness and heat fuming and steaming may also result in vomiting and diarrhea. This may compound the situation by leading to a sudden and substantial loss of liquids through vomiting and diarrhea. Therefore, damp heat may result in oral thirst through any of three mechanisms. If dampness is predominant, there will be thirst but less desire to drink. If heat or vomiting and diarrhea are predominant, there will be thirst with a stronger desire to drink.

Treatment based on pattern discrimination:

I. External contraction of wind heat[6]

---

[6] In clinical practice, thirst is an important symptom for the differentiation of the external contraction of wind. Absence of thirst is not necessarily a symptom of wind cold. But presence of thirst is always a symptom of wind heat or exterant cold with internal heat.

Symptoms: Thirst, fever with either no or inhibited sweating, slight aversion to wind and cold, headache, cough, sore throat, a red tongue tip with thin, white or thin, yellow fur, and a floating, rapid pulse

Therapeutic principles: Resolve the exterior with acrid, cool agents, clear heat and resolve toxins

Acupuncture & moxibustion:

Chi Ze (Lu 5) *Qu Ze* (Per 3)	Together, these points clear heat and engender liquids.
He Gu (LI 4) *Wai Guan* (TB 5)	Together, these points clear heat and resolve the exterior.
Shao Shang (Lu 11)	Clears heat and resolve toxins

Additions & subtractions: For headache in the temples, add *Tai Yang* (M-HN-9). For headache in the forehead, add *Yin Tang* (M-HN-3). And for headache in the occipital region, add *Feng Chi* (GB 20).

Chinese medicinal formula: *Yin Qiao San* (Lonicera & Forsythia Powder)

Ingredients: Flos Lonicerae Japonicae (*Jin Yin Hua*), 9g, Fructus Forsythiae Suspensae (*Lian Qiao*), 9g, uncooked Radix Platycodi Grandiflori (*Jie Geng*), 6g, Herba Menthae Haplocalysis (*Bo He*), 3g, Folium Bambusae (*Zhu Ye*), 9g, Radix Glycyrrhizae (*Gan Cao*), 3g, Herba Schizonepetae Tenuifoliae (*Jing Jie*), 3g, warm Semen Praeparatus Sojae (*Dan Dou Chi*), 6g, uncooked Fructus Arctii Lappae (*Niu Bang Zi*), 9g, Rhizoma Phragmitis Communis (*Lu Gen*), 12g

Additions & subtractions: If thirst is severe, add Radix Trichosanthis Kirlowii (*Tian Hua Fen*), 9g. If there is heat damaging the fluids, add uncooked Radix Rehmanniae (*Sheng Di*), 9g, and Tuber Ophiopogonis Japonici (*Mai Men Dong*), 9g. If heat invades the lungs with cough, asthma, and severe thirst, use *Ma Xing Shi Gan Tang* (Ephedra, Apricot Kernel, Licorice & Gypsum Decoction) : uncooked Herba Ephedrae (*Ma*

Huang), 3g, Semen Pruni Armeniacae (*Xing Ren*), 6g, uncooked Gypsum Fibrosum (*Shi Gao*), 18g, Radix Glycyrrhizae (*Gan Cao*), 6g.

2. *Yang ming* channel heat

Symptoms: Great thirst with strong desire for profuse drink, great fever, great sweating, and a surging, large, forceful pulse

Therapeutic principles: Clear heat and engender liquids

Acupuncture & moxibustion:

Ye Men (TB 2)	Together, these points engender liquids to quench
Zhao Hai (Ki 6)	the thirst.
Cheng Jiang (CV 24)	

Li Dui (St 45)	Together, these points clear heat when pricked to
Shang Yang (LI 1)	induce bleeding.

Additions & subtractions: For severe thirst and profuse sweating, add *Zu San Li* (St 36) to boost the qi and help engender liquids.

Chinese medicinal formula: *Bai Hu Tang* (White Tiger Decoction)

Ingredients: Uncooked Gypsum Fibrosum (*Shi Gao*), 30g, uncooked Rhizoma Anemarrhenae Asphodeloidis (*Zhi Mu*), 9g, Radix Glycyrrhizae (*Gan Cao*), 6g, Semen Oryzae Sativae (*Geng Mi*), 9g

Additions & subtractions: If great fever and great sweating damage qi and yin, add white Radix Panacis Ginseng (*Bai Ren Shen*), 6g, or Radix Panacis Quinguifolii (*Xi Yang Shen*), 6g.

3. *Yang ming* bowel repletion

Symptoms: Thirst with desire for chilled drinks, fever, red eyes, vexation and agitation, constipation, glomus in the stomach and abdomen, abdominal pain that refuses pressure, yellow urine, yellow, dry tongue fur, and a deep, replete, forceful pulse

Therapeutic principles: Greatly precipitate heat binding

Acupuncture & moxibustion:

Fu Liu (Ki 7)	Engenders liquids to quench the thirst
Li Dui (St 45) *Shang Yang* (LI 1)	Together, these points drain heat when pricked to induce bleeding.
Tian Shu (St 25) *Shang Ju Xu* (St 37)	Together, these points precipitate heat binding.

Additions & subtractions: For severe heat binding, add *Zhi Gou* (TB 6). For severe thirst, add *Zhao Hai* (Ki 6).

Chinese medicinal formula: *Da Cheng Qi Tang* (Major Order the Qi Decoction)

Ingredients: Uncooked Radix Et Rhizoma Rhei (*Da Huang*), 12g, Mirabilitum (*Mang Xiao*), 9g, uncooked Fructus Immaturus Citri Aurantii (*Zhi Shi*), 12g, ginger mix-fried Cortex Magnoliae Officinalis (*Hou Po*), 15g

4. Heat entering the constructive division

Symptoms: Thirst with little desire to drink or even no thirst, fever worse at night, vexation with reduced sleep, clouded spirit and delirium, faintly visible macules and papules in some cases, a crimson, dry tongue, and a fine, rapid pulse

Therapeutic principles: Clear the constructive and nourish yin

Acupuncture & moxibustion:

Shi Xuan (M-UE-1)	When pricked to bleed (7-10 drops of the blood at each point), drains heat and arouses the spirit
San Yin Jiao (Sp 6) *Tai Xi* (Ki 3)	Together, these points clear the constructive and nourish yin to quench thirst.

Chinese medicinal formula: Modified *Qing Ying Tang* (Clear the Constructive Decoction)

Ingredients: Cornu Bubali (*Shui Niu Jiao*), 20g, uncooked Radix Rehmanniae (*Sheng Di*), 15g, Radix Scrophulariae Ningpoensis (*Xuan Shen*), 9g, Folium Bambusae (*Zhu Ye*), 9g, Tuber Ophiopogonis Japonici (*Mai Men Dong*), 9g, Radix Salviae Miltiorrhizae (*Dan Shen*), 6g, uncooked Rhizoma Coptidis Chinensis (*Huang Lian*), 6g, Flos Lonicerae Japonicae (*Jin Yin Hua*), 9g, Fructus Forsythiae Suspensae (*Lian Qiao*), 6g

Note: Because Cornu Rhinocerotis (*Xi Jiao*) is from an endangered species, we have substituted Cornu Bubali (water buffalo horn) routinely in all instances where it appears as a standard ingredient of a standard formula.

5. Heat entering the blood division

Symptoms: Dry mouth or thirst but no desire to swallow water after washing the mouth with it, blood ejection, nosebleed, bloody stool, purple or black macules, delirium or mania, vexation and pain in the chest, a subjective feeling of abdominal fullness, bloody stool which is easy to discharge, a crimson tongue, and a deep, replete, forceful pulse

Therapeutic principles: Clear heat and resolve toxins, cool the blood and dispel stasis

Acupuncture & moxibustion:

Shi Xuan (M-UE-1)	Drains heat and resolves toxins when pricked to let 7-10 drops of the blood
Da Ling (Per 7) *Ren Zhong* (GV 26)	Together, these points clear the heart and quiet the spirit.
He Gu (LI 4) *San Yin Jiao* (Sp 6)	Together, these points cool the blood and dispel the stasis to stop bleeding.

Chinese medicinal formula: Modified *Xi Jiao Di Huang Tang* (Rhinoceros Horn & Rehmannia Decoction)

Ingredients: Cornu Bubali (*Shui Niu Jiao*), 20g, uncooked Radix Rehmanniae (*Sheng Di*), 30g, uncooked Radix Rubrus Paeoniae Lactiflorae (*Chi Shao*), 12g, Cortex Radicis Moutan (*Dan Pi*), 9g, uncooked Radix Scutellariae Baicalensis (*Huang Qin*), 9g, uncooked Radix Et Rhizoma Rhei (*Da Huang*), 6g

6. Summer-heat damaging the liquids

Symptoms: Thirst with desire to drink, fever, vexation, sweating, short voidings of dark-colored urine, fatigue, reduced qi, a red tongue, and a vacuous, rapid pulse

Therapeutic principles: Clear summer-heat and boost the qi, nourish yin and engender liquids

Acupuncture & moxibustion:

Jin Jin Yu Ye (M-HN-20)	Engenders liquids (prick to bleed)
Qu Ze (Per 3) *Wei Zhong* (Bl 40)	Together, these points clear summer-heat (prick to bleed).
Zu San Li (St 36) *San Yin Jiao* (Sp 6)	Together, these points boost the qi and nourish yin.

Chinese medicinal formula: *Qing Shu Yi Qi Tang* (Clear Summer-heat & Boost the Qi Decoction)

Ingredients: Radix Panacis Qinquefolii (*Xi Yang Shen*), 6g, Herba Dendrobii (*Shi Hu*), 9g, Tuber Ophiopogonis Japonici (*Mai Men Dong*), 9g, uncooked Rhizoma Coptidis Chinensis (*Huang Lian*), 3g, Folium Bambusae (*Zhu Ye*), 6g, Petiolus Nelumbinis Nuciferae (*He Geng*), 15g, uncooked Rhizoma Anemarrhenae Asphodeloidis (*Zhi Mu*), 6g, Radix Glycyrrhizae (*Gan Cao*), 3g, Semen Oryzae Sativae (*Geng Mi*), 15g, Pericarpium Citrulli Vulgaris (*Xi Gua Pi*), 20g

7. Dryness damaging the liquids

Symptoms: Thirst, vexation, fever, headache, a dry cough with no phlegm, dry nose and throat, a dry tongue with reduced fur, and a vacuous, big, rapid pulse

Therapeutic principles: Clear dryness and moisten the lungs

Acupuncture & moxibustion:

He Gu (LI 4)	Together, these points clear dryness and resolve
Qu Chi (LI 11)	the exterior.
San Yin Jiao (Sp 6)	Together, these points moisten the lungs and
Fei Shu (Bl 13)	engender liquids to quench thirst.

Additions & subtractions: For severe dry cough, add *Lie Que* (Lu 7) and *Fu Liu* (Ki 7).

Chinese medicinal formula: *Qing Zao Jiu Fei Tang* (Clear Dryness & Rescue the Lungs Decoction)

Ingredients: Honey mix-fried Folium Mori Albi (*Sang Ye*), 9g, uncooked Gypsum Fibrosum (*Shi Gao*), 12g, uncooked Radix Codonopsitis Pilosulae (*Dang Shen*), 6g, Radix Glycyrrhizae (*Gan Cao*), 3g, Semen Lini (*Hu Ma Ren*), 6g, Gelatinum Corii Asini (*E Jiao*), 6g, Tuber Ophiopogonis Japonici (*Mai Men Dong*), 6g, Semen Pruni Armeniacae (*Xing Ren*), 6g, Folium Eriobotryae Japonicae (*Pi Pa Ye*), 6g

8. Exuberant internal heat

Symptoms: Thirst with a desire to drink, great fever, vexation and agitation, confused speech, insomnia, astringent voidings of dark-colored urine, blood ejection, nosebleed, eruption of macules, a red tongue with yellow fur, and a rapid, forceful pulse

Therapeutic principles: Drain fire and resolve toxins

Acupuncture & moxibustion:

Shi Xuan (M-UE-1)	Drains fire and resolves toxins when pricked to bleed
Nei Guan (Per 6) *Yong Quan* (Ki 1) *Nei Ting* (St 44)	Together, these points drain fire and lead the heat downward to quiet the spirit and stop bleeding.
San Yin Jiao (Sp 6) *Tai Xi* (Ki 3)	Together, these points nourish yin to quench thirst.

Additions & subtractions: For a persistent high fever, add *Da Zhui* (GV 14) and *Wei Zhong* (BI 40).

Chinese medicinal formula: *Huang Lian Jie Du Tang* (Coptis Resolve Toxins Decoction)

Ingredients: Uncooked Rhizoma Coptidis Chinensis (*Huang Lian*), 6g, uncooked Radix Scutellariae Baicalensis (*Huang Qin*), 6g, uncooked Cortex Phellodendri (*Huang Bai*), 6g, uncooked Fructus Gardeniae Jasminoidis (*Zhi Zi*), 9g

9. Yin vacuity with effulgent fire

Symptoms: Thirst and dry throat which are worse at night, dizziness, tinnitus, steaming bone tidal fever, vexatious heat in the five hearts, pain and weakness of the low back and knees, insomnia, night sweats, a red tongue with reduced fur, and a fine, rapid pulse

Therapeutic principles: Enrich yin and downbear fire

Acupuncture & moxibustion:

Fei Shu (Bl 13) *Pi Shu* (Bl 20) *Wei Shu* (Bl 21)	Together, these points nourish yin and engender liquids.

Tai Xi (Ki 3)	Together, these points enrich yin and downbear
Ran Gu (Ki 2)	fire.
San Yin Jiao (Sp 6)	

Additions & subtractions: For severe dizziness and tinnitus, add *Yong Quan* (Ki 1) to lead effulgent fire downward. For insomnia, add *Shen Men* (Ht 7).

Chinese medicinal formula: Modified *Zhi Bai Di Huang Wan* (Anemarrhena & Phellodendron Rehmannia Pills)

Ingredients: Prepared Radix Rehmanniae (*Shu Di*), 18g, uncooked Radix Dioscoreae Oppositae (*Shan Yao*), 12g, steamed Fructus Corni Officinalis (*Shan Zhu Yu*), 12g, Sclerotium Poriae Cocos (*Fu Ling*), 6g, salt mix-fried Rhizoma Alismatis (*Ze Xie*), 6g, Cortex Radicis Moutan (*Dan Pi*), 9g, salt mix-fried Rhizoma Anemarrhenae Asphodeloidis (*Zhi Mu*), 9g, salt mix-fried Cortex Phellodendri (*Huang Bai*), 6g, Tuber Ophiopogonis Japonici (*Mai Men Dong*), 9g

I0. Insufficiency of stomach yin (mainly seen in wasting & thirsting disease)

Symptoms: Thirst with profuse drinking, frequent and profuse urination, fatigue, shortness of breath, and a vacuous, fine, forceless pulse

Therapeutic principles: Boost the qi and engender fluids, moisten dryness and allay thirst

Acupuncture & moxibustion:

Lie Que (Lu 7)	Together, these points moisten dryness and
Zhao Hai (Ki 6)	engender fluids.

Fei Shu (Bl 13)	Together, these points nourish yin.
Pi Shu (Bl 20)	
Wei Shu (Bl 21)	

Zu San Li (St 36)	Boosts the qi and helps engender fluids

Additions & subtractions: For dizziness and tinnitus, add *Qu Chi* (LI 11) and *Tai Xi* (Ki 3) to nourish yin and clear heat.

Chinese medicinal formula: *Yu Ye Tang* (Jade Fluids Decoction)

Ingredients: Uncooked Radix Dioscoreae Oppositae (*Shan Yao*), 30g, stir-fried Radix Astragali Membranacei (*Huang Qi*), 15g, uncooked Rhizoma Anemarrhenae Asphodeloidis (*Zhi Mu*), 15g, Endothelium Corneum Gigeriae Galli (*Ji Nei Jin*), 6g, uncooked Radix Puerariae (*Ge Gen*), 9g, uncooked Fructus Schisandrae Chinensis (*Wu Wei Zi*), 9g, Radix Trichosanthis Kirlowii (*Tian Hua Fen*), 9g

II. Yin vacuity coupled with external contraction

Symptoms: Thirst with desire to drink, heart vexation, possible fever, headache, and slight aversion to wind and cold, scanty or no sweating, sore throat, a red tongue, and a wiry, rapid pulse

Therapeutic principles: Enrich yin and resolve the exterior

Acupuncture & moxibustion:

He Gu (LI 4)   Together, these points resolve the exterior.
Wai Guan (TB 5)

Fu Liu (Ki 7)   Together, these points enrich yin.
Tai Xi (Ki 3)

Additions & subtractions: For high fever, add *Da Zhui* (GV 14) and *Qu Chi* (Lu 11).

Chinese medicinal formula: Modified *Wei Rui Tang* (Polygonatum Odoratum Decoction)

Ingredients: Rhizoma Polygonati Odorati (*Yu Zhu*), 9g, Bulbus Allii Fistulosi (*Cong Bai*), 6g, Radix Platycodi Grandiflori (*Jie Geng*), 6g, Radix Cynanchi Baiwai (*Bai Wai*), 3g, warm Semen Praeparatus Sojae

(*Dan Dou Chi*), 9g, Herba Menthae Haplocalysis (*Bo He*), 3g, mix-fried Radix Glycyrrhizae (*Zhi Gan Cao*), 3g

12. Water rheum collecting internally

Symptoms: Thirst with no desire to drink, ejection (*i.e.*, vomiting) of water immediately after taking it in, a dry tongue, borborygmus, encumbered limbs, vomiting of foamy drool, cold form (*i.e.*, body) and limbs, minor edema in the face, chest oppression, pain in the lateral costal regions exacerbated by coughing, possible fever and headache, inhibited urination, white tongue fur, and a wiry pulse

Therapeutic principles: Disinhibit water and penetrate dampness, warm yang and transform qi

Acupuncture & moxibustion:

Yin Ling Quan (Sp 6) *Shui Fen* (CV 9)	Together, these points disinhibit water and penetrate dampness.
Qi Hai (CV 6) *Zu San Li* (St 36)	Together, these points boost the qi to distribute fluids.
Fu Liu (Ki 7)	Warms kidney yang and transforms qi to disinhibit water

Additions & subtractions: For fever, add *Zhi Zheng* (SI 7) and *Feng Men* (Bl 12). For headache, add *Tai Yang* (M-HN-9) and *Yin Tang* (M-HN-3).

Chinese medicinal formula: *Wu Ling San* (Five [Ingredient] Poria Powder)

Ingredients: Sclerotium Polypori Umbellati (*Zhu Ling*), 9g, Rhizoma Alismatis (*Ze Xie*), 15g, uncooked Rhizoma Atractylodis Macrocephalae (*Bai Zhu*), 9g, Sclerotium Poriae Cocos (*Fu Ling*), 9g, Ramulus Cinnamomi Cassiae (*Gui Zhi*), 6g

13. Water rheum collecting internally coupled with vacuous heat

Symptoms: Thirst with desire for scanty drink, vomiting of clear drool, encumbered limbs, cough with foamy expectoration, minor edema of the eyelids and face, borborygmus, vexation and insomnia, dry stool, inhibited voiding of yellow urine, possible fever, yellow or white tongue fur, and a wiry, rapid pulse

Therapeutic principles: Foster yin, clear heat, and disinhibit water

Acupuncture & moxibustion:

Yin Ling Quan (Sp 9) *Shui Fen* (CV 9)	Together, these points disinhibit water.
San Yin Jiao (Sp 6) *Zu San Li* (St 36)	Together, these points disinhibit dampness, protect and foster yin.
Zhao Hai (Ki 6)	Fosters kidney yin and clears vacuous heat

Additions & subtractions: For vexation and insomnia, add *Shen Mai* (Bl 62).

Chinese medicinal formula: *Zhu Ling Tang* (Polyporum Umbellatum Decoction)

Ingredients: Sclerotium Polypori Umbellati (*Zhu Ling*), 9g, Rhizoma Alismatis (*Ze Xie*), 9g, Sclerotium Poriae Cocos (*Fu Ling*), 9g, Gelatinum Corii Asini (*E Jiao*), 9g, Talcum (*Hua Shi*), 9g

14. Water binding with heat

Symptoms: Thirst and dry tongue, hardness and fullness between the heart and lower abdomen that refuses pressure, constipation, slight tidal fever in the afternoon, and a deep, tight, forceful pulse

Therapeutic principles: Drain heat and expel water

Acupuncture & moxibustion:

Shui Dao (St 28)   Together, these points expel water.
Shui Fen (CV 9)

Tian Shu (St 25)   Together, these points free the stools to drain heat
Shang Ju Xu (St 37)   and expel water.

Nei Ting (St 44)   Drains heat

Chinese medicinal formula: *Da Xian Xiong Tang* (Major Sinking into the Chest Decoction)

Ingredients: Uncooked Radix Et Rhizoma Rhei (*Da Huang*), 9g, Mirabilitum (*Mang Xiao*), 9g, Radix Euphorbiae Kansui (*Gan Sui*), 1g (powdered and taken with the strained decoction)

15. Spleen-stomach qi vacuity

Symptoms: Thirst with desire for warm drinks, reduced qi with disinclination to speak, possible fever, spontaneous sweating, fatigue and weakness of the limbs, a bright, white facial complexion, loose stools, possible prolapses of the rectum and uterus in some cases, thin, white tongue fur, and a vacuous pulse

Therapeutic principles: Supplement the center and boost the qi

Acupuncture & moxibustion:

Da Du (Sp 2)   Together, these points supplement the center and
Zu San Li (St 36)   boost the qi.

Qi Hai (CV 6)   Together, these points warm yang and transform
Shen Que (CV 8)   qi to distribute fluids.

Bai Hui (GV 20)   Upbears the qi to help the spleen distribute fluids

Note: Use moxibustion on all the above points.

Chinese medicinal formula: *Bu Zhong Yi Qi Tang* (Supplement the Center & Boost the Qi Decoction)

Ingredients: Honey stir-fried Radix Astragali Membranacei (*Huang Qi*), 15g, mix-fried Radix Glycyrrhizae (*Zhi Gan Cao*), 6g, honey stir-fried Radix Codonopsitis Pilosulae (*Dang Shen*), 9g, bran stir-fried Rhizoma Atractylodis Macrocephalae (*Bai Zhu*), 9g, stir-fried Radix Angelicae Sinensis (*Dang Gui*), 9g, stir-fried Pericarpium Citri Reticulatae (*Chen Pi*), 6g, honey mix-fried Rhizoma Cimicifugae (*Sheng Ma*), 3g, stir-fried Radix Bupleuri (*Chai Hu*), 3g

16. Blood stasis

Symptoms: Thirst with desire to drink but without desire to swallow the water after washing the mouth with it, a soot black facial complexion, scaly skin, prominent veins, crab-claw markings (*i.e.*, spider nevi), dysmenorrhea and menstruation with purple, black clots in women, a bluish purple tongue and lips, and a fine and choppy, bound, or regularly interrupted pulse

Therapeutic principles: Move and nourish the blood

Acupuncture & moxibustion:

He Gu (LI 4)	Together, these points move the qi and quicken
San Yin Jiao (Sp 6)	the blood to transform blood stasis.
Xue Hai (Sp 10)	Together, these points nourish and quicken the
Ge Shu (Bl 17)	blood to transform blood stasis.
Pi Shu (Bl 20)	

Chinese medicinal formula: Modified *Tong Qiao Huo Xue Tang* (Free the Portals & Quicken the Blood Decoction)

Ingredients: Wine mix-fried Radix Rubrus Paeoniae Lactiflorae (*Chi Shao*), 9g, wine mix-fried Radix Ligustici Wallichii (*Chuan Xiong*), 9g, wine mix-fried Radix Angelicae Sinensis (*Dang Gui*), 9g, Flos Carthami Tinctorii (*Hong Hua*), 6g, uncooked Semen Pruni Persicae (*Tao Ren*), 9g, uncooked Radix Rehmanniae (*Sheng Di*), 9g, uncooked Rhizoma Zingiberis (*Sheng Jiang*), 3g, Fructus Zizyphi Jujubae (*Da Zao*), 3 pieces

17. Damp heat fuming & steaming

Symptoms: Thirst with desire to drink, vexation and agitation, fatigue, poor appetite, glomus and oppression in the chest and stomach, abdominal pain, cramping when there is vomiting and diarrhea, inhibited defecation, thick, dry, yellow tongue fur, and a soggy, rapid pulse

Therapeutic principles: Clear heat and disinhibit dampness, upbear the clear and downbear the turbid

Acupuncture & moxibustion:

Zhong Wan (CV 12)	Together, these points upbear the clear and
Tian Shu (St 25)	downbear the turbid.
Shang Ju Xu (St 37)	
Zu San Li (St 36)	

Nei Ting (St 44)	Together, these points clear heat and disinhibit
Yin Ling Quan (Sp 9)	dampness.

Chinese medicinal formula: *Can Shi Tang* (Excrementum Bombicis Decoction)

Ingredients: Excrementum Bombicis Batryticati (*Can Sha*), 15g, Semen Coicis Lachryma-jobi (*Yi Yi Ren*), 15g, Semen Germinatus Sojae (*Dou Juan*), 12g, Fructus Chaenomalis Lagenariae (*Mu Gua*), 9g, Rhizoma Coptidis Chinensis (*Huang Lian*), 6g, clear Rhizoma Pinelliae Ternatae (*Ban Xia*), 6g, Radix Scutellariae Baicalensis (*Huang Qin*), 6g, Medulla Tetrapanacis Papyriferi (*Tong Cao*), 3g, Fructus Gardeniae Jasminoidis (*Zhi Zi*), 6g, processed Fructus Evodiae Rutecarpae (*Wu Zhu Yu*), 1g

10
Drooling from the Corner of the Mouth
(*Kou Jiao Liu Xian*)

This refers to saliva flowing from the corner of the mouth involuntarily.

Disease causes, disease mechanisms:

1. External wind attacking the network vessels

Wind is a yang evil and is, therefore, likely to attack the upper body. If wind attacks the face and enters the network vessels there, it may block the vessels leading to loss of nourishment of the sinews therein. If nourishment is insufficient, the sinews will become relaxed or slack. Thus, the lips will fail to contain liquids and fluids in the mouth and hence drooling from the corner of the mouth occurs.

2. Wind & phlegm exiting above

Phlegm may be the result of spleen vacuity which fails to move and transport water dampness, or it can be due to a constitution with abiding phlegm. Wind may be due to yin vacuity from aging, enduring disease, and sexual taxation where yin fails to check yang properly. If wind drafts and discharges phlegm upward, phlegm may lodge in and block the network vessels and deprive the sinews of sufficient nourishment. This then leads to relaxation or slackening of the sinews. If this happens to the lips, the lips will fail to contain the saliva and thus there will be drooling. If the wind and phlegm are discharged upward and cloud the clear portals, such drooling will be accompanied by essence spirit (*i.e.*, mental-emotional) problems.

3. Spleen-stomach heat steaming

Spleen-stomach heat can be due to a constitutional brewing of heat or from addiction to rich, fatty foods and alcohol. Brewing and then steaming, this heat can force liquids out into the mouth in an increased amount. Therefore, drooling occurs.

4. Spleen vacuity failing to contain

Spleen vacuity can arise from constitutional vacuity, dietary irregularities, enduring disease, or over-thinking. The spleen governs movement and transformation. Therefore, if the spleen becomes vacuous, water dampness will tend to accumulate. Since the spleen also governs the muscles, if there is spleen vacuity, the muscles will receive less nourishment, leading to the muscles becoming weak. Thus the lips may fail to contain liquids in the mouth. With more liquid and less containment, drooling is due to occur.

In addition, worm accumulation and mouth sores in children can respectively lead to stomach disharmony and make children try to avoid swallowing their saliva so as to avoid pain. This may also lead to drooling.

Treatment based on pattern discrimination:

I. External wind attacking the network vessels

Symptoms: Sudden drooling from the corner of the mouth on the affected side, facial numbness and tingling, deviated mouth and eyes, inability to close the eye properly, aversion to wind and cold, lacrimation, white tongue fur, and a floating, wiry pulse

Therapeutic principles: Dispel wind and unblock the network vessels

Acupuncture & moxibustion:

Di Cang (St 4)	Together, these points dispel wind from the local
Jia Che (St 6)	area and unblock the network vessels so as to contain the fluids and stop drooling. Use connecting method from *Di Cang* to *Jia Che*.

He Gu (LI 4)	Together, these points dispel wind and resolve the
Wai Guan (TB 5)	exterior.

Additions & subtractions: For tearing of the eyes, add *Zan Zhu* (Bl 2). For fever, add *Qu Chi* (LI 11).

Chinese medicinal formula: Modified *Qian Zheng San* (Lead to the Symmetry Powder)

Ingredients: Rhizoma Typhonii Gigantei (*Bai Fu Zi*), 9g, Bombyx Batryticatus (*Jiang Can*), 9g, Periostracum Cicadae (*Chan Tui*), 12g, Buthus Martensi (*Quan Xie*), 6g, Radix Ledebouriellae Divaricatae (*Fang Feng*), 6g, Ramulus Uncariae Cum Uncis (*Gou Teng*), 9g

Note: In clinical practice, this pattern primarily describes Bell's palsy.

2. Wind & phlegm exiting above

Symptoms: Persistent drooling, tinnitus, vexation, hemiplegia with numbness and tingling, deviated mouth and eyes, deviated tongue with inhibited speech, possible lack of clarity of the essence spirit (*i.e.*, mind), dizziness, vertigo, a gurgling sound of phlegm in the throat, thick, slimy tongue fur, and a wiry, slippery pulse

Therapeutic principles: Extinguish wind, level the liver, and subdue yang

Acupuncture & moxibustion:

Di Cang (St 4)	Together, these points unblock the network vessels
Jia Che (St 6)	in the local area and contain the fluids. Use
Cheng Jiang (CV 24)	connecting method from *Di Cang* to *Jia Che*.

Tai Chong (Liv 3)	Together, these points level the liver, subdue
Tai Xi (Ki 3)	yang, and transform phlegm.
Feng Long (St 40)	

Additions and subtractions: For lack of clarity of the essence spirit, add *Ren Zhong* (GV 26) and *Su Liao* (GV 25). For deviated mouth and eyes, refer to "Deviated Mouth & Eyes" in Volume 1 (p. 135-42). For hemiplegia, depending upon the affected part of the body, select from: *Ji Quan* (Ht 1), *Chi Ze* (Lu 5), *He Gu* (LI 4), *Jian Yu* (LI 15), *Qu Chi* (LI 11), and *Wai Guan* (TB 5) if the upper limb is affected; *Ba Xie* (M-UE-22) if the hand is affected; *Wei Zhong* (Bl 40), *Yang Ling Quan* (GB 34), *San Yin Jiao* (Sp 6), *Jie Xi* (St 41), *Qiu Xu* (GB 40), and *Zhao Hai* (Ki 6) if the lower limb is affected; and *Tong Li* (Ht 5) and *Jin Jin* (M-HN-20b) *Yu Ye* (M-HN-20a) if the tongue is affected and/or the speech inhibited.

Chinese medicinal formula: Modified *Ding Xian Wan* (Stabilize Seizure Pills)

Ingredients: Stir-fried till yellow Rhizoma Gastrodiae Elatae (*Tian Ma*), 12g, Bulbus Fritillariae Cirrhosae (*Chuan Bei Mu*), 6g, lime-processed Rhizoma Pinelliae Ternatae (*Ban Xia*), 9g, Sclerotium Poriae Cocos (*Fu Ling*), 9g, Sclerotium Pararadicis Poriae Cocos (*Fu Shen*), 9g, processed Rhizoma Arisaematis (*Tian Nan Xing*), 9g, Rhizoma Acori Graminei (*Shi Chang Pu*), 6g, Radix Glycyrrhizae (*Gan Cao*), 3g, uncooked Bombyx Batryticatus (*Jiang Can*), 9g, Succinum (*Hu Po*), 1g (powder & take with the strained decoction), Medulla Junci Effusi (*Deng Xin Cao*), 3g, Pericarpium Citri Reticulatae (*Chen Pi*), 6g, licorice-processed Radix Polygalae Tenuifoliae (*Yuan Zhi*), 6g, Cortex Radicis Moutan (*Dan Pi*), 9g

Note: This formula is taken after the acute stage. It treats the root of the disease. In clinical practice, this pattern primarily describes the sequelae of windstroke or apoplexy.

3. Phlegm heat exiting above

Symptoms: Drooling, deviated mouth and eyes, inhibited speech, hemiplegia with numbness and tingling, headache, vertigo, tinnitus, phlegm rales in the throat, a red tongue with yellow, slimy tongue fur, and a slippery, rapid pulse

Therapeutic principles: Clear heat and transform phlegm, extinguish wind and unblock the network vessels

Acupuncture & moxibustion:

Di Cang (St 4)	See above
Jia Che (St 6)	
Cheng Jiang (CV 24)	
Feng Long (St 40)	Together, these points clear heat and transform
Nei Ting (St 44)	phlegm.
Xing Jian (Liv 2)	Together, these points clear heat and extinguish
Yong Quan (Ki 1)	wind to unblock the network vessels.

Chinese medicinal formula: Modified *Tian Ma Gou Teng Yin* (Gastrodia & Uncaria Drink)

Ingredients: Stir-fried till yellow Rhizoma Gastrodiae Elatae (*Tian Ma*), 12g, Ramulus Uncariae Cum Uncis (*Gou Teng*), 12g, Radix Achyranthis Bidentatae (*Niu Xi*), 6g, Concha Haliotidis (*Shi Jue Ming*), 15g, Ramulus Loranthi Seu Visci (*Sang Ji Sheng*), 6g, Fructus Gardeniae Jasminoidis (*Zhi Zi*), 9g, uncooked Radix Scutellariae Baicalensis (*Huang Qin*), 9g, Sclerotium Pararadicis Poriae Cocos (*Fu Shen*), 9g, bile-processed Rhizoma Arisaematis (*Dan Nan Xing*), 9g, lime-processed Rhizoma Pinelliae Ternatae (*Ban Xia*), 9g, Concretio Silicea Bambusae (*Tian Zhu Huang*), 9g, uncooked Bombyx Batryticatus (*Jiang Can*), 9g, Bulbus Fritillariae Cirrhosae (*Chuan Bei Mu*), 6g

Note: This pattern primarily describes the sequelae of windstroke or apoplexy.

4. Spleen-stomach heat steaming

Symptoms: Drooling from the corners of the mouth, a worrying tongue (*i.e.*, constant, restless licking of the lips), mouth sores, bad breath, vexatious thirst, reduced food intake, constipation, dark-colored urine, easy hungering, dry lips, a red tongue with yellow or yellow, slimy fur, and a slippery, rapid pulse

Therapeutic principles: Clear and drain spleen-stomach heat

Acupuncture & moxibustion:

Di Cang (St 4)   See above
Jia Che (St 6)
Cheng Jiang (CV 24)
Lian Quan (CV 23)

He Gu (LI 4)   Together, these points clear and transform spleen-
Zu San Li (St 36)   stomach dampheat.
Yin Ling Quan (Sp 9)

Chinese medicinal formula: Modified *Xie Huang San* (Drain the Yellow Powder)

Ingredients: Herba Agastachis Seu Pogostemi (*Huo Xiang*), 12g, Radix Ledebouriellae Divaricatae (*Fang Feng*), 6g, uncooked Fructus Gardeniae Jasminoidis (*Zhi Zi*), 6g, uncooked Gypsum Fibrosum (*Shi Gao*), 15g, Radix Glycyrrhizae (*Gan Cao*), 6g, uncooked Radix Rehmanniae (*Sheng Di*), 9g, Cortex Radicis Moutan (*Dan Pi*), 6g

5. Spleen vacuity failing to contain

Symptoms: Drooling of clear, thin saliva, reduced food intake, poor appetite, distention and fullness in the abdomen, sloppy diarrhea, a bright, white facial complexion, reduced qi with no inclination to speak, a pale tongue with thin, white fur, and a deep, weak pulse

Therapeutic principles: Fortify the spleen and boost the qi

Acupuncture & moxibustion:

Cheng Jiang (CV 24)   Together, these points contain fluids.
Da Ying (St 5)

Zhong Wan (CV 12)	Together, these points fortify the spleen and
Guan Yuan (CV 4)	supplement the qi.
Zu San Li (St 36)	
San Yin Jiao (Sp 6)	

Chinese medicinal formula: Modified *Liu Jun Zi Tang* (Six Gentlemen Decoction)

Ingredients: Rice stir-fried Radix Codonopsitis Pilosulae (*Dang Shen*), 9g, bran stir-fried Rhizoma Atractylodis Macrocephalae (*Bai Zhu*), 6g, Sclerotium Poriae Cocos (*Fu Ling*), 6g, mix-fried Radix Glycyrrhizae (*Zhi Gan Cao*), 3g, uncooked Rhizoma Zingiberis (*Sheng Jiang*), 6g, dry Rhizoma Zingiberis (*Gan Jiang*), 3g, stir-fried Pericarpium Citri Reticulatae (*Chen Pi*), 6g, lime-processed Rhizoma Pinelliae Ternatae (*Ban Xia*), 6g

Note: This pattern is most often seen in infants and young children. However, it may also be seen in the elderly.

6. Roundworm accumulation in children

Symptoms: Drooling from both corners of the mouth, a dull, yellow facial complexion with white mucus in some cases, emaciation, pain around the navel which sometimes gets worse and sometimes gets better (*i.e.*, is episodic and paroxysmal), irregular defecation, flowery, peeling tongue fur, and white macules or papules on the inside of the lips

Therapeutic principles: Warm the organs and calm the roundworms

Acupuncture & moxibustion:

Zhong Wan (CV 12)	Together, these points warm the center and
Da Heng (Sp 15)	harmonize the stomach to stop drooling.
Zu San Li (St 36)	

Nei Guan (Per 6)	Together, these points soothe the center and
Gong Sun (Sp 4)	downbear the qi, quiet and dispel the roundworms.

Bai Chong Wo   An extra-channel empirical point for expelling
(M-LE-34)   roundworms

Chinese medicinal formula: *Wu Mei Wan* (Mume Pills)

Ingredients: Uncooked Fructus Pruni Mume (*Wu Mei*), 9g, Radix Codonopsitis Pilosulae (*Dang Shen*), 6g, Herba Asari Cum Radice (*Xi Xin*), 3g, uncooked Cortex Phellodendri (*Huang Bai*), 6g, processed Radix Lateralis Praeparatus Aconiti Carmichaeli (*Fu Zi*), 3g, stir-fried Ramulus Cinnamomi Cassiae (*Gui Zhi*), 3g, uncooked Rhizoma Coptidis Chinensis (*Huang Lian*), 6g, dry Rhizoma Zingiberis (*Gan Jiang*), 6g, uncooked Radix Angelicae Sinensis (*Dang Gui*), 6g, Pericarpium Zanthoxyli Bungeani (*Chuan Jiao*), 3g

Note: This pattern is, in actuality, a combination of vacuity and repletion, hot and cold. Parasites and worms typically occur when the righteous qi, in this case the spleen qi, is vacuous. Accumulation of dampness transforms into heat; so there is damp heat. This is the environment in which parasites or worms are engendered. Because children's spleens are inherently immature and, therefore, weak, they are most at risk for worm infestation. The above formula is extremely effective when there is flowery, peeling tongue fur.

II
Mouth Sores (*Kou Chuang*)

Mouth sores refer to ulcerations of the lips, tongue, and the other parts inside the mouth.

Disease causes, disease mechanisms:

I. Heat accumulated in the heart & spleen

Addiction to rich, fatty, acrid food may transform heat, leading to heat accumulation in the heart and spleen. The spleen opens into the portal of the mouth, while the heart opens into the tongue. If accumulated heat steams and flames upward along the channels to the mouth, this heat may burn and putrefy the flesh there. As a result, mouth sores occur.

2. Non-interaction between the heart & kidneys

Constitutional vacuity, unrestrained sexual activity, enduring disease, and aging can all cause kidney yin vacuity. Kidney yin is supposed to check heart yang and maintain the proper balance between heart fire and kidney water. If yin becomes vacuous, kidney yin may fail in that function and heart fire may subsequently become exuberant. Out of control, heart fire may flame upward into the mouth along the channels, burning and damaging the flesh there and thus leading to the arising of sores in the mouth.

Treatment based on pattern discrimination:

I. Heat accumulated in the heart & spleen

Symptoms: Bright red sores in the mouth and on the tongue which is swollen and painful, swollen cheeks and/or gums which affect food intake, in some severe cases, thirst with a liking for chilled drinks, yellow urine, constipation, a red tongue with yellow fur, and a rapid pulse

Therapeutic principles: Clear heat and drain fire

Acupuncture & moxibustion:

Xin Shu (Bl 15)   Together, these points clear heat and drain fire.
Pi Shu (Bl 20)
Xiao Chang Shu (Bl 27)
Yin Ling Quan (Sp 9)
Lao Gong (Per 8)

Chinese medicinal formulas:

Orally: Modified *Liang Ge San* (Cool the Diaphragm Powder)

Ingredients: Fructus Forsythiae Suspensae (*Lian Qiao*), 9g, uncooked Radix Et Rhizoma Rhei (*Da Huang*), 6g, Mirabilitum (*Mang Xiao*), 6g, stir-fried Rhizoma Anemarrhenae Asphodeloidis (*Zhi Mu*), 6g, wine stir-fried Rhizoma Coptidis Chinensis (*Huang Lian*), 6g, Herba Menthae Haplocalysis (*Bo He*), 3g, Folium Bambusae (*Zhu Ye*), 9g, Radix Glycyrrhizae (*Gan Cao*), 6g, uncooked Rhizoma Cimicifugae (*Sheng Ma*), 6g

Topically: *Fu Yan San* (Go to the Banquet Powder)

Ingredients: Uncooked Radix Scutellariae Baicalensis (*Huang Qin*), 15g, uncooked Rhizoma Coptidis Chinensis (*Huang Lian*), 15g, uncooked Fructus Gardeniae Jasminoidis (*Zhi Zi*), 15g, dry Rhizoma Zingiberis (*Gan Jiang*), 15g, uncooked Cortex Phellodendri (*Huang Bai*), 15g , Herba Asari Cum Radice (*Xi Xin*), 15g

Method of use: Powder the above medicinals, mix together, and apply to the affected area(s).

2. Non-interaction between the heart & kidneys

Symptoms: Sores in the mouth and tongue with frequent recurrence, pale color on the sore surface, vexation, insomnia, vexatious heat in the five hearts, a red tongue with reduced fur, and a fine, rapid pulse

Therapeutic principles: Enrich yin and downbear fire

Acupuncture & moxibustion:

Zhao Hai (Ki 6)   Together, these points relieve pain.
Lian Quan (CV 23)

Yong Quan (Ki 1)   Together, these points enrich yin, downbear fire,
San Yin Jiao (Sp 6)   and restore the interaction between the heart and
Tai Xi (Ki 3)   kidneys.
Nei Guan (Per 6)

Additions & subtractions: For night sweats, add *Yin Xi* (Ht 6).

Chinese medicinal formulas:

Orally: Modified *Zhi Bai Di Huang Wan* (Anemarrhena & Phellodendron Rehmannia Pills)[7]

Ingredients: Prepared Radix Rehmanniae (*Shu Di*), 12g, uncooked Radix Dioscoreae Oppositae (*Shan Yao*), 6g, steamed Fructus Corni Officinalis (*Shan Zhu Yu*), 6g, Sclerotium Poriae Cocos (*Fu Ling*), 6g, salt mix-fried Rhizoma Alismatis (*Ze Xie*), 6g, Cortex Radicis Moutan (*Dan Pi*), 12g, salt mix-fried Rhizoma Anemarrhenae Asphodeloidis (*Zhi Mu*), 9g, salt

---

[7] If the result of this formula is slow, we can add Cortex Cinnamomi Cassiae (*Rou Gui*), 1-2g. Cinnamon, in this case, returns yang back to its lower origin. This one, simple modification can greatly enhance the effects of this formula. However, one should remember that Cinnamon should only be decocted for five minutes and one should be sure to use the real Cortex Cinnamomi Cassiae (usually expensive) and not the common Cinnamon (*Gui Pi*) which is usually cheap.

mix-fried Cortex Phellodendri (*Huang Bai*), 9g, Radix Scrophulariae Ningpoensis (*Xuan Shen*), 9g

Topically: *Kou Chuang San* (Mouth Sores Powder)

Ingredients: Uncooked Cortex Phellodendri (*Huang Bai*), 15g , Pulvis Indigonis (*Qing Dai*), 15g, Cortex Cinnamomi Cassiae (*Rou Gui*), 15g, Borneol (*Bing Pian*), 10g

Method of use: Powder the above medicinals, mix together, and apply to the affected area(s).

12
Copious Spittle (*Duo Tuo*)

This refers to a symptom where the patient feels like spitting out the saliva from their mouth due to the fact or subjective sensation that excessive saliva is engendered.

Disease causes, disease mechanisms:

1. Kidney vacuity & water spilling over

Constitutional vacuity, congenital insufficiency, and enduring diseases can lead to kidney yang depletion. "The kidneys governs water" and "Spittle is the humor of the kidneys." If there is kidney yang vacuity or depletion, the kidneys cannot warm and transform water. This then gives rise to water spilling over and ascending. Therefore, copious spittle with frequent spitting may occur.

2. Spleen-stomach vacuity cold

Excessive consumption of raw or chilled foods may damage the spleen, leading to spleen-stomach vacuity cold. It is also possible for the spleen and stomach to be constitutionally vacuous and cold. With spleen-stomach vacuity cold, devitalized spleen yang will give rise to failure of movement and transformation. This then may result in water dampness spilling over and ascending. Therefore, frequent spitting occurs.

3. Lung qi vacuity cold

Enduring cough and asthma may consume the qi and damage yang or damage to lung yin may reach (*i.e.*, affect) yang. As a result, there may be lung qi vacuity cold. If there is lung qi vacuity cold, the qi will fail to transform liquids, and thus copious spittle with frequent spitting will occur.

Treatment based on pattern discrimination:

I. Kidney vacuity & water spilling over

Symptoms: Copious saliva and frequent spitting, dizziness, tinnitus, heart palpitations, shortness of breath exacerbated on exertion, in severe cases, palpitations around the umbilicus, a pale tongue with white, slippery fur, and a wiry, slippery pulse

Therapeutic principles: Warm yang and disinhibit water

Acupuncture & moxibustion:

Qi Hai (CV 6) Together, when moxaed, these points warm yang.
Guan Yuan (CV 4)

Qi Hai Shu (Bl 24) Use these points alternatively with the above
Ming Men (GV 6) group.
Guan Yuan Shu (Bl 26)

Fu Liu (Ki 7) Warms the kidneys and disinhibits the water

Chinese medicinal formula: Modified *Zhen Wu Tang* (True Warrior Decoction)

Ingredients: Bland Radix Lateralis Praeparatus Aconiti Carmichaeli (*Fu Zi*), 6g, uncooked Rhizoma Atractylodis Macrocephalae (*Bai Zhu*), 9g, Radix Albus Paeoniae Lactiflorae (*Bai Shao*), 6g, uncooked Rhizoma Zingiberis (*Sheng Jiang*), 9g, Sclerotium Poriae Cocos (*Fu Ling*), 9g, salt stir-fried Radix Morindae Officinalis (*Ba Ji Tian*), 6g, Semen Plantaginis (*Che Qian Zi*), 6g, Fructus Lycii Chinensis (*Gou Qi Zi*), 6g

2. Spleen-stomach vacuity cold

Symptoms: Copious saliva and frequent spitting, poor appetite, loose stools, reduced qi with disinclination to speak, fatigue and lack of strength, a pale, fatty, tender, and teeth-marked tongue with white, slimy fur, and a soggy pulse

Therapeutic principles: Warm the spleen and dissipate cold

Acupuncture & moxibustion:

Zhong Wan (CV 12)	Together, when moxaed, these points warm the
Shen Que (CV 8)	spleen and dissipate cold.
Guan Yuan (CV 4)	
Zu San Li (St 36)	
Gong Sun (Sp 4)	

Chinese medicinal formula: *Li Zhong Wan* (Rectify the Center Pills)

Ingredients: Honey stir-fried Radix Codonopsitis Pilosulae (*Dang Shen*), 6g, dry Rhizoma Zingiberis (*Gan Jiang*), 6g, mix-fried Radix Glycyrrhizae (*Zhi Gan Cao*), 6g, bran stir-fried Rhizoma Atractylodis Macrocephalae (*Bai Zhu*), 9g

Additions & subtractions: If there is spleen-kidney yang vacuity, add bland Radix Lateralis Praeparatus Aconiti Carmichaeli (*Fu Zi*), 6g. If there is spleen vacuity with damp encumbrance manifest by sliminess in the mouth, fullness and oppression in the stomach and abdomen, diarrhea, heavy-headedness, etc., use Modified *Dao Gong San* (Abduct the Result Powder): Rice stir-fried Radix Codonopsitis Pilosulae (*Dang Shen*), 9g, Sclerotium Poriae Cocos (*Fu Ling*), 9g, mix-fried Radix Glycyrrhizae (*Zhi Gan Cao*), 6g, bran stir-fried Rhizoma Atractylodis Macrocephalae (*Bai Zhu*), 9g, stir-fried Pericarpium Citri Reticulatae (*Chen Pi*), 9g, Semen Coicis Lachryma-jobi (*Yi Yi Ren*), 20g, Rhizoma Atractylodis (*Cang Zhu*), 6g, stir-fried Semen Dolichori Lablab (*Bai Bian Dou*), 12g.

Note: This pattern is frequently seen after an acute episode of infantile convulsions.

3. Lung qi vacuity cold

Symptoms: Frequent spitting of foamy saliva, no thirst, possible enuresis, frequent urination, vertigo, qi shortage not enough for breathing, fatigued spirit and lack of strength, reduced food intake, cold form, a pale tongue, and a vacuous, weak pulse

Therapeutic principles: Warm and boost the lung qi

Acupuncture & moxibustion:

Shan Zhong (CV 17)   Together, these points warm lung qi.
Qi Hai (CV 6)

Gao Huang (Bl 43)   Together, when moxaed, these points warm the
Fei Shu (Bl 13)   lungs.
Guan Yuan Shu (Bl 26)

Chinese medicinal formula: Modified *Gan Cao Gan Jiang Tang* (Licorice & Dry Ginger Decoction)

Ingredients: Mix-fried Radix Glycyrrhizae (*Zhi Gan Cao*), 12g, dry Rhizoma Zingiberis (*Gan Jiang*), 6g, honey stir-fried Radix Codonopsitis Pilosulae (*Dang Shen*), 9g, stir-fried Ramulus Cinnamomi Cassiae (*Gui Zhi*), 6g, Fructus Zizyphi Jujubae (*Da Zao*), 4 pieces

13
Crimson Lips (*Chun Jiang*)

Crimson lips refers to lips which are deep red, looking purplish red or dull purplish.

Disease causes, disease mechanisms:

Spleen-stomach replete heat fuming & steaming

Excessive consumption of fatty, sweet, rich, acrid food may lead to heat accumulation in the spleen and stomach. "The spleen's efflorescence is in the lips." If replete heat fumes and steams, the lips will become crimson.

Treatment based on pattern discrimination:

Spleen-stomach replete heat fuming & steaming

Symptoms: Crimson, purplish lips, mouth and tongue sores, dry mouth with desire for chilled drinks, constipation, voidings of yellow, dark-colored urine, a red tongue with yellow fur, and a slippery, rapid pulse

Therapeutic principles: Clear heat and drain fire

Acupuncture & moxibustion:

Shang Yang (LI 1) *Li Dui* (St 45)	Together, these points drain heat when pricked to bleed.
Nei Ting (St 44) *Jie Xi* (St 41) *Yin Ling Quan* (Sp 9)	Together, these points clear and drain spleen-stomach heat.

Chinese medicinal formula: *Xie Huang Tang* (Drain the Yellow Decoction)

Ingredients: Herba Agastachis Seu Pogostemi (*Huo Xiang*), 9g, Fructus Gardeniae Jasminoidis (*Zhi Zi*), 9g, Gypsum Fibrosum (*Shi Gao*), 20g, Radix Glycyrrhizae (*Gan Cao*), 6g, Radix Ledebouriellae Divaricatae (*Fang Feng*), 6g

14
Cyanotic Lips (*Chun Qing Zi*)

This refers to lips which are green-blue and purplish in color.

Disease causes, disease mechanisms:

Cyanotic lips are often encountered in serious diseases. Generally speaking, they are mainly due to stasis (blood stasis and phlegm stasis), heat, and/or cold involving the viscera of the lungs, heart, kidneys, liver, and spleen.

1. Lung heat

This heat mainly comes from warm heat evils that have entered the body via the mouth and nose or from other external evils that enter the body and then transform into heat. Heat is a yang evil which, therefore, damages liquids. Blood and liquids share a common source. If liquids are damaged, the blood will become condensed. Subsequently, the qi and blood will congest and stagnate. In that case, cyanotic lips are the reflection of that congestion and stagnation.

2. Phlegm turbidity blocking the lungs

"The spleen is the source of phlegm production, while the lungs are the place where phlegm is stored." Spleen vacuity not moving and transforming water dampness is often the cause of phlegm turbidity blocking the lungs. Once blocked by phlegm turbidity, the lungs will fail to diffuse and downbear, leading to disharmony of the vessels since, "The lungs face the hundreds of vessels." As a result, qi and blood become static and blocked and cyanotic lips will occur. If this phlegm turbidity transforms into heat over time, cyanotic lips will be accompanied by signs of heat.

3. Qi stagnation & blood stasis

Qi stagnation and blood stasis may be both the cause and result of one another. Any factor that causes qi stagnation may lead to blood stasis and vice versa.

In most cases, liver depression and qi stagnation is to blame. The liver governs coursing and discharge. If emotional disturbance and frustration cause lack of coursing and discharge, this will lead to liver depression and qi stagnation. This, in turn, will affect the movement of the qi and blood. In that case, blood stasis will occur, blocking the channels and network vessels and leading to cyanotic lips.

"The heart governs the blood and vessels" and thus the heart is often also to blame for blood stasis. Aging, a weak constitution, or enduring disease can cause blood stasis which then leads to blockage of the heart vessels. When heart vessels are blocked, the blood will not move normally and thus there are cyanotic lips.

"The spleen is the source of qi and blood engenderment and transformation." The spleen may become vacuous due to a constitutional vacuity, enduring disease, and/or dietary irregularities. If there is spleen vacuity, less qi and blood will be engendered. Being vacuous, qi cannot move the blood normally, while, also being vacuous, the blood cannot transform enough qi to move the blood. As a result, blood stasis will occur and block the vessels. Therefore, there will be cyanotic lips.

4. *Shao yin* vacuity cold

Vacuity cold may be due to constitutional vacuity, enduring disease, or aging. If external evils enter the body, they may transform into cold when they enter the interior, thus leading to yin cold exuberance in the interior and life gate fire depletion. "Cold is associated with congealing and contraction." In such cases, water liquids and the blood will not be moved properly. Therefore, there are cyanotic lips.

Treatment based on pattern discrimination:

I. Lung heat

Symptoms: Cyanotic lips, cough and panting with rapid breathing, flaring nostrils, gaping mouth and raised shoulders, unresolved fever, thirst, sweating, thin, yellow tongue fur, and a slippery, rapid pulse

Therapeutic principles: Diffuse and drain the lungs with acrid, cool agents and calm panting

Acupuncture & moxibustion:

Fei Shu (Bl 13)	Together, these points diffuse and drain the lungs.
Da Zhui (GV 14)	
He Gu (LI 4)	
Kong Zui (Lu 6)	

Shao Shang (Lu 11)	Together, these points drain replete heat.
Nei Ting (St 44)	

Chinese medicinal formula: *Ma Xing Shi Gan Tang* (Ephedra, Apricot Kernel, Licorice & Gypsum Decoction)

Ingredients: Uncooked Herba Ephedrae (*Ma Huang*), 5g, Semen Pruni Armeniacae (*Xing Ren*), 9g, uncooked Gypsum Fibrosum (*Shi Gao*), 20g, Radix Glycyrrhizae (*Gan Cao*), 6g

Additions & subtractions: If heat damages the fluids, add honey stir-fried Cortex Radicis Mori Albi (*Sang Bai Pi*), 9g, Rhizoma Phragmitis Communis (*Lu Gen*), 9g, and stir-fried Rhizoma Anemarrhenae Asphodeloidis (*Zhi Mu*), 9g.

2. Phlegm heat blocking the lungs

Symptoms: Cyanotic lips, cough with yellow phlegm which is difficult to expectorate, dry cough with rapid breathing, glomus and oppression in the chest and diaphragm, short voidings of dark-colored urine, a red tongue with yellow, slimy fur, and a slippery, rapid pulse

Therapeutic principles: Clear heat and transform phlegm, downbear qi and stop the cough

Acupuncture & moxibustion:

Yu Zhong (Ki 26) *Yun Men* (Lu 2) *Shi Men* (CV 5)	Together, these points clear heat, downbear qi, and stop the cough.
Da Zhui (GV 14) *Fei Shu* (Bl 13) *Feng Long* (St 40)	Together, these points clear heat and transform phlegm.

Chinese medicinal formula: *Qing Qi Hua Tan Wan* (Clear the Qi & Transform Phlegm Pills)

Ingredients: Fructus Trichosanthis Kirlowii (*Gua Lou*), 9g, uncooked Pericarpium Citri Reticulatae (*Chen Pi*), 9g, uncooked Radix Scutellariae Baicalensis (*Huang Qin*), 9g, Semen Pruni Armeniacae (*Xing Ren*), 9g, uncooked Fructus Immaturus Citri Aurantii (*Zhi Shi*), 9g, Sclerotium Poriae Cocos (*Fu Ling*), 9g, bile-processed Rhizoma Arisaematis (*Dan Nan Xing*), 12g, lime-processed Rhizoma Pinelliae Ternatae (*Ban Xia*), 12g

3. Cold phlegm blocking the lungs

Symptoms: Cyanotic lips, coughing and panting with phlegm rales which can be triggered by exposure to cold, glomus and fullness in the chest and diaphragm, inability to lie flat or there will be dyspnea, a white, lusterless facial complexion, a pale tongue with white, slimy fur, and a slippery pulse

Therapeutic principles: Dissipate cold and flush away phlegm

Acupuncture & moxibustion:

Chi Ze (Lu 5) *Lie Que* (Lu 7)	Together, these points free the qi flow of the lung channel.

Tian Tu (CV 22)	Together, these points downbear qi and stop *Shan*
Zhong (CV 17)	cough.

Feng Long (St 40)	Together, these points warm and dissipate cold
and *Fei Shu* (Bl 13)	flush away phlegm when moxa is burnt on the
Feng Men (Bl 12)	head of the needle.

Chinese medicinal formula: *Leng Xiao Wan* (Chilly Wheezing Pills)

Ingredients: Uncooked Herba Ephedrae (*Ma Huang*), 30g, Radix Lateralis Praeparatus Aconiti Carmichaeli (*Fu Zi*), 30g, Herba Asari Cum Radice (*Xi Xin*), 30g, Pericarpium Zanthoxyli Bungeani (*Chuan Jiao*), 30g, Alumen (*Ming Fan*), 30g, Fructus Gleditschiae Chinensis (*Zao Jiao*), 30g, Rhizoma Pinelliae Ternatae (*Ban Xia*), 30g, bile-processed Rhizoma Arisaematis (*Dan Nan Xing*), 30g, Semen Pruni Armeniacae (*Xing Ren*), 30g, Radix Glycyrrhizae (*Gan Cao*), 30g, Radix Asteris Tatarici (*Zi Wan*), 60g, Flos Tussilaginis Farfarae (*Kuan Dong Hua*), 60g

Method of use: Make a paste with ginger juice and the powder of the above Chinese medicinals. Take about 6g each day and apply topically to *Fei Shu* (Bl 13) and *Feng Men* (Bl 12). Keep this paste on all day.

4. Qi stagnation & blood stasis

Symptoms: Cyanotic lips, fullness and stabbing pain in the chest; in severe cases, pain in the chest radiating to the upper back or pain in the upper back radiating to the chest; panting and cough with expectoration, inability to lie flat, a dull tongue with possible static macules, and a wiry, choppy pulse

Therapeutic principles: Move the qi and transform phlegm, quicken the blood and dispel stasis

Acupuncture & moxibustion:

He Gu (LI 4)	Together, these points move the qi, quicken the
San Yin Jiao (Sp 6)	blood, and dispel stasis.

Zhong Fu (Lu 1)   Together, these points rectify the qi, transform
Feng Long (St 40)   phlegm, and stop the cough.

Additions & subtractions: For pain in the chest radiating to the upper back, add *Shan Zhong* (CV 17) and *Ge Shu* (Bl 17).

Chinese medicinal formula: *Gua Lou Xie Bai Ban Xia Tang* (Trichosanthes Fruit, Chinese Chive & Pinellia Decoction) plus *Shi Xiao San* (Loose a Smile Powder)

Ingredients: Fructus Trichosanthis Kirlowii (*Gua Lou*), 6g, Bulbus Allii (*Xie Bai*), 6g, lime-processed Rhizoma Pinelliae Ternatae (*Ban Xia*), 9g, uncooked Semen Pruni Persicae (*Tao Ren*), 9g, Flos Carthami Tinctorii (*Hong Hua*), 9g, Pollen Typhae (*Pu Huang*), 9g, vinegar stir-fried Feces Trogopterori Seu Pteromi (*Wu Ling Zhi*), 6g, Lignum Dalbergiae Odoriferae (*Jiang Xiang*), 9g, Fructus Citri Aurantii (*Zhi Ke*), 6g

Additions & subtractions: If blood stasis is severe, add wine mix-fried Radix Rubrus Paeoniae Lactiflorae (*Chi Shao*), 9g, wine mix-fried Radix Ligustici Wallichii (*Chuan Xiong*), 9g, and wine mix-fried Radix Angelicae Sinensis (*Dang Gui*), 9g.

5. Liver qi depression & binding

Symptoms: Cyanotic lips, a bluish grey facial complexion, chest oppression and shortage of qi, distention and fullness of the lateral costal regions, reduced food intake and torpid intake, frequent sighing, a dull tongue with thin, white fur, and a wiry, soggy pulse

Therapeutic principles: Course the liver, rectify qi, and quicken the blood

Acupuncture & moxibustion:

Ri Yue (GB 24)   Together, these points course the liver and rectify
Qi Men (Liv 14)   the qi.
Tai Chong (Liv 3)

Ge Shu (Bl 17)	Together, these points move the qi and quicken
Gan Shu (Bl 18)	the blood.

Additions & subtractions: For torpid intake, add *Zhong Wan* (CV 12).

Chinese medicinal formula: *Xiao Yao San* (Rambling Powder)

Ingredients: Radix Bupleuri (*Chai Hu*), 6g, bran stir-fried Rhizoma Atractylodis Macrocephalae (*Bai Zhu*), 9g, uncooked Radix Albus Paeoniae Lactiflorae (*Bai Shao*), 9g, wine mix-fried Radix Angelicae Sinensis (*Dang Gui*), 9g, Sclerotium Poriae Cocos (*Fu Ling*), 6g, Herba Menthae Haplocalysis (*Bo He*), 3g, mix-fried Radix Glycyrrhizae (*Zhi Gan Cao*), 3g, uncooked Rhizoma Zingiberis (*Sheng Jiang*), 3g

6. Qi vacuity & scanty blood

Symptoms: Cyanotic lips, a withered yellow facial complexion, fatigued spirit and lack of strength, reduced qi with disinclination to speak, heart palpitations and racing heart, impaired memory, insomnia, a pale tongue with white fur, and a vacuous, weak pulse

Therapeutic principles: Boost the qi and supplement the blood, fortify the spleen and nourish the heart

Acupuncture & moxibustion:

Xin Shu (Bl 15)	Together, these points supplement the blood.
Ge Shu (Bl 17)	
Pi Shu (Bl 20)	

Tai Yuan (Lu 9)	Together, these points boost the qi, supplement the
Xue Hai (Sp 10)	blood, and quicken the blood.
Zu San Li (St 36)	

Chinese medicinal formula: Modified *Gui Pi Tang* (Return the Spleen Decoction)

Ingredients: Honey stir-fried Radix Astragali Membranacei (*Huang Qi*), 15g, bran stir-fried Rhizoma Atractylodis Macrocephalae (*Bai Zhu*), 9g, stir-fried Radix Angelicae Sinensis (*Dang Gui*), 12g, Arillus Euphoriae Longanae (*Long Yan Rou*), 6g, Sclerotium Pararadicis Poriae Cocos (*Fu Shen*), 3g, Radix Auklandiae Lappae (*Mu Xiang*), 3g, mix-fried Radix Glycyrrhizae (*Zhi Gan Cao*), 3g, Radix Codonopsitis Pilosulae (*Dang Shen*), 9g, prepared Radix Rehmanniae (*Shu Di*), 6g, Radix Albus Paeoniae Lactiflorae (*Bai Shao*), 9g

Additions & subtractions: If there is insomnia, add Semen Zizyphi Spinosae (*Suan Zao Ren*), 9g, and licorice-processed Radix Polygalae Tenuifoliae (*Yuan Zhi*), 9g. If there are heart palpitations and a bound or regularly interrupted pulse, use *Zhi Gan Cao Tang* (Mix-fried Licorice Decoction): Mix-fried Radix Glycyrrhizae (*Zhi Gan Cao*), 12g, uncooked Rhizoma Zingiberis (*Sheng Jiang*), 9g, Radix Panacis Ginseng (*Ren Shen*), 6g, uncooked Radix Rehmanniae (*Sheng Di*), 15g, stir-fried Ramulus Cinnamomi Cassiae (*Gui Zhi*), 9g, Gelatinum Corii Asini (*E Jiao*), 6g, Tuber Ophiopogonis Japonici (*Mai Men Dong*), 9g, Semen Cannabis Sativae (*Huo Ma Ren*), 6g, Fructus Zizyphi Jujubae (*Da Zao*), 5 pieces.

7. Cold striking the *shao yin*

Symptoms: Cyanotic lips, a somber or even soot-black facial complexion, fear of cold and cold limbs, panting on exertion, spontaneous sweating, low back and knee soreness and weakness, a pale, fat tongue with glossy fur, and a deep, tight pulse

Therapeutic principles: Warm the kidneys and dissipate cold

Acupuncture & moxibustion:

Shen Que (CV 8) *Guan Yuan* (CV 4)	Together, when moxaed, these points warm yang and dissipate cold.
Shen Shu (Bl 23) *Ming Men* (GV 4) *Guan Yuan Shu* (Bl 26)	Together, when moxaed, these points warm the kidneys, assist yang, and dissipate cold.

Chinese medicinal formula: *Si Ni Tang* (Four Counterflows Decoction)

Ingredients: Bland Radix Lateralis Praeparatus Aconiti Carmichaeli (*Fu Zi*), 6g, dry Rhizoma Zingiberis (*Gan Jiang*), 9g, mix-fried Radix Glycyrrhizae (*Zhi Gan Cao*), 6g

15
Pale White Lips (*Chun Dan Bai*)

Pale white lips are lips which are bloodless or faintly colored.

Disease causes, disease mechanisms:

1. Blood vacuity

Blood vacuity may be the result of a) constructive qi insufficiency which fails to transform the blood, b) constitutional insufficiency, c) spleen-stomach vacuity which fails to engender and transform the blood, d) bleeding due to spleen vacuity which fails to contain the blood or to traumatic injury, or e) enduring disease or over-thinking which consumes the blood insidiously day by day. Once vacuous, the blood cannot nourish the flesh and skin. Therefore, the lips turn pale.

2. Spleen qi vacuity

Spleen qi vacuity may be due to dietary irregularities or enduring disease. If there is spleen qi vacuity, the clear yang will not be upborne, while the turbid yin will not be downborne. This leads to water spilling over into the flesh and skin, resulting in undernourishment of the flesh and skin. Pale lips may occur as a result.

Treatment based on pattern discrimination:

I. Blood vacuity

Symptoms: Pale lips, a white, lusterless or withered yellow facial complexion, lusterless nails, heart palpitations, vexation, insomnia, dizziness and flowery (*i.e.*, blurred) vision, scanty, pale colored and/or delayed menstruation or amenorrhea in women, a pale tongue with white fur, and a fine, forceless pulse

Therapeutic principles: Nourish the blood and harmonize the constructive

Acupuncture & moxibustion:

Zhong Wan (CV 12)   Together, these points fortify the spleen and
Zu San Li (St 36)   engender the blood.
San Yin Jiao (Sp 6)

Xin Shu (Bl 15)   Together, these points nourish the blood and
Ge Shu (Bl 17)   harmonize the constructive.
Pi Shu (Bl 20)

Additions & subtractions: For menstrual problems, add *Guan Yuan* (CV 4) and *Gan Shu* (Bl 18).

Chinese medicinal formula: Modified *Gui Pi Tang* (Return the Spleen Decoction)

Ingredients: Honey stir-fried Radix Astragali Membranacei (*Huang Qi*), 15g, bran stir-fried Rhizoma Atractylodis Macrocephalae (*Bai Zhu*), 9g, stir-fried Radix Angelicae Sinensis (*Dang Gui*), 12g, Arillus Euphoriae Longanae (*Long Yan Rou*), 6g, Sclerotium Pararadicis Poriae Cocos (*Fu Shen*), 3g, Radix Auklandiae Lappae (*Mu Xiang*), 3g, mix-fried Radix Glycyrrhizae (*Zhi Gan Cao*), 3g, Radix Codonopsitis Pilosulae (*Dang Shen*), 9g, prepared Radix Rehmanniae (*Shu Di*), 6g, Radix Albus Paeoniae Lactiflorae (*Bai Shao*), 9g

2. Spleen qi vacuity

Symptoms: Pale, lusterless lips, a withered, white facial complexion, fatigue and lack of strength, expectoration of foamy drool, vomiting, glomus and oppression in the stomach and abdomen, a pale tongue with white fur, and a deep, weak pulse

Acupuncture & moxibustion:

Shen Que (CV 8)	Together, when moxaed, these points boost the qi.
Qi Hai (CV 6)	
Guan Yuan (CV 4)	

Da Du (Sp 2)	Together, when moxaed, these points fortify the
Zu San Li (St 36)	spleen and harmonize the stomach.
Zhong Wan (CV 12)	

Additions & subtractions: For dizziness and headache, add *Bai Hui* (GV 20). For loose stools, add *Tian Shu* (St 25).

Chinese medicinal formula: *Xiang Sha Liu Jun Zi Tang* (Aucklandia & Amomum Six Gentlemen Decoction)

Ingredients: Rice stir-fried Radix Codonopsitis Pilosulae (*Dang Shen*), 9g, bran stir-fried Rhizoma Atractylodis Macrocephalae (*Bai Zhu*), 9g, Sclerotium Poriae Cocos (*Fu Ling*), 6g, mix-fried Radix Glycyrrhizae (*Zhi Gan Cao*), 6g, stir-fried Pericarpium Citri Reticulatae (*Chen Pi*), 6g, lime-processed Rhizoma Pinelliae Ternatae (*Ban Xia*), 9g, uncooked Radix Auklandiae Lappae (*Mu Xiang*), 6g, Fructus Amomi (*Sha Ren*), 3g

16
Cracked Dry Lips (*Chun Zao Lie*)

Cracked dry lips here refers to lips with narrow fissures in them due to lack of moisture.

Disease causes, disease mechanisms:

I. Replete fire in the upper burner

Replete fire may be the result of contraction of external evils which enter the body and transform into fire or from excesses of the five affects which transform fire and mutually enflame heart fire. Fire is a yang evil; so its nature is that it consumes liquids. If fire consumes so much liquid that the lips receive less moisture, there will be cracked dry lips.

2. Replete spleen-stomach heat

Replete spleen and stomach heat may arise from addiction to sweet, fatty, rich, greasy food or from evils entering the body and transforming into heat. When heat is exuberant, it consumes much liquid. Thus the lips receive less moisture, and hence the lips are cracked and dry.

3. Yin vacuity, fire effulgence

Yin vacuity, fire effulgence may be due to replete heat damaging yin or to enduring consumption of yin due to chronic disease or unrestrained sexual activity. If yin vacuity, fire effulgence steams upward, the lips will become dry and cracked.

4. Stomach yin insufficiency

This insufficiency may be the result of chronic disease which consumes stomach yin, late stage yin humor damage due to febrile disease, or addiction to acrid food. The lips are associated with the spleen and stomach. When there is stomach yin vacuity, the lips will suffer from insufficient moistening, and thus the lips will become cracked and dry.

Treatment based on pattern discrimination

I. Replete fire in the upper burner

Symptoms: Dry, cracked lips, fever, thirst, a red face, vexatious heat in the chest and diaphragm, mouth and tongue sores, constipation, dark-colored urine, possible sore throat, blood ejection and spontaneous external bleeding (*i.e.*, epistaxis and hemoptysis), a red tongue with yellow fur, and a slippery, rapid pulse

Therapeutic principles: Drain fire and free the stools, clear the upper burner and discharge the lower

Acupuncture & moxibustion:

Cheng Jiang (CV 24)   Engenders fluids to moisten the lips

Wai Guan (TB 5)   Together, these points drain heat in the upper
Guan Chong (TB 1)   burner (prick *Guan Chong* and *Shao Shang* to
Shao Shang (Lu 11)   bleed).

Shang Ju Xu (St 37)   Together, these points free the stools to drain the
Tian Shu (St 25)   fire.

Additions & subtractions: For fever, add *He Gu* (LI 4) and *Qu Chi* (LI 11). For hot flashes in the face, add *Nei Ting* (St 44).

Chinese medicinal formula: *Liang Ge San* (Cool the Diaphragm Powder)

Ingredients: Fructus Forsythiae Suspensae (*Lian Qiao*), 12g, uncoooked Radix Et Rhizoma Rhei (*Da Huang*), 9g, Mirabilitum (*Mang Xiao*), 6g, Fructus Gardeniae Jasminoidis (*Zhi Zi*), 9g, Radix Scutellariae Baicalensis (*Huang Qin*), 9g, Herba Menthae Haplocalysis, (*Bo He*), 6g, Folium Bambusae (*Zhu Ye*), 6g, Radix Glycyrrhizae (*Gan Cao*) 3g

2. Replete spleen-stomach heat

Symptoms: Red, swollen, cracked, dry lips, dry mouth, thirst with drinking a lot of chilled drinks, profuse food intake with easy hunger, possible bad breath, constipation, a red tongue with yellow fur, and a surging, rapid, forceful or deep, replete pulse

Therapeutic principles: Clear and drain replete spleen-stomach heat

Acupuncture & moxibustion:

Zhi Gou (TB 6)	Frees the channel qi flow of the three burners
He Gu (LI 4) *Qu Chi* (LI 11)	Together, these points clear heat in the *yang ming* channel.
Shang Ju Xu (St 37) *Nei Ting* (St 44)	Together with *Zhi Gou*, these points drain heat in the bowels.

Additions & subtractions: For clamoring stomach, add *Fu Liu* (Ki 7).

Chinese medicinal formula: Modified *Qing Wei San* (Clear the Stomach Powder)

Ingredients: Uncooked Gypsum Fibrosum (*Shi Gao*), 30g, wine stir-fried Rhizoma Coptidis Chinensis (Huang Lian), 6g, uncooked Radix Rehmanniae (*Sheng Di*), 12g, uncooked Radix Angelicae Sinensis (*Dang Gui*), 6g, Cortex Radicis Moutan (*Dan Pi*), 9g, uncooked Rhizoma Cimicifugae (*Sheng Ma*), 6g, uncooked Radix Et Rhizoma Rhei (*Da Huang*), 6g

Additions & subtractions: If heat damages spleen and stomach fluids, add Tuber Ophiopogonis Japonici (*Mai Men Dong*), 9g, and Radix Glehniae Littoralis (*Sha Shen*), 9g.

3. Yin vacuity, fire effulgence

Symptoms: Red, cracked, dry lips, red cheekbones, dry mouth, tidal fever, night sweats, vacuity vexation, insomnia, constipation, dark-colored urine, a red tongue with reduced fur, and a fine, rapid pulse

Therapeutic principles: Enrich yin and clear heat

Acupuncture & moxibustion:

Cheng Jiang (CV 24) Engenders fluids to moisten the lips

Zhao Hai (Ki 6) Together, these points enrich yin and clear heat.
Tai Xi (Ki 3)

San Yin Jiao (Sp 6) Together, these points clear heat in the yin
Fu Liu (Ki 7) division.

Additions & subtractions: For night sweats, add *Yin Xi* (Ht 6). For seminal emission, add *Zhi Shi* (Bl 52). For vexation and insomnia, add *Shen Men* (Ht 7).

Chinese medicinal formula: Modified *Zi Yin Di Huang Wan* (Nourish Yin Rehmannia Pills)

Ingredients: Prepared Radix Rehmanniae (*Shu Di*), 18g, stir-fried Radix Dioscoreae Oppositae (*Shan Yao*), 12g, steamed Fructus Corni Officinalis (*Shan Zhu Yu*), 12g, Fructus Schisandrae Chinensis (*Wu Wei Zi*), 6g, Tuber Ophiopogonis Japonici (*Mai Men Dong*), 6g, uncooked Radix Angelicae Sinensis (*Dang Gui*), 6g, Flos Chrysanthemi Morifolii (*Ju Hua*), 6g, Fructus Lycii Chinensis (*Gou Qi*), 9g, stir-fried Semen Zizyphi Spinosae (*Suan Zao Ren*), 9g

4. Stomach yin insufficiency

Symptoms: Cracked, dry lips, dry mouth, hunger without desire for food, possible hiccup and dry vomiting, a red tongue with reduced fur, and a fine, rapid pulse

Therapeutic principles: Nourish the stomach and engender liquids

Acupuncture & moxibustion:

Cheng Jiang (CV 24) Engenders fluids to moisten the lips

Zhong Wan (CV 12) Together, these points nourish and harmonize the
Nei Guan (Per 6) stomach.

Wei Shu (Bl 21) Together, these points fortify the spleen and
Pi Shu (Bl 20) nourish the stomach to engender fluids.

Additions & subtractions: If the above formula does not work very well, change *Wei Shu* and *Pi Shu* to *Tai Xi* (Ki 3) and *Fu Liu* (Ki 7).

Chinese medicinal formula: *Zi Chun Yin* (Nourish the Lips Drink)

Ingredients: Uncooked Radix Rehmanniae (*Sheng Di*), 9g, Herba Dendrobii (*Shi Hu*), 12g, Caulis Bambusae In Taeniis (*Zhu Ru*), 6g, uncooked Gypsum Fibrosum (*Shi Gao*), 15g, Radix Angelicae Sinensis (*Dang Gui*), 9g, Radix Albus Paeoniae Lactiflorae (*Bai Shao*), 9g, Radix Glycyrrhizae (*Gan Cao*), 6g

Remarks: As a local treatment in addition to the above, use of the popular Chinese ointment *Jing Wan Hong* (Ten Million Ten Thousand Reds) is very effective. This medicine is a bit messy, but it is very good for cracked, dry lips. Apply directly to the lips two time per day.

17
Lip Tremor (*Chun Chan Dong*)

Lip tremor refers to involuntarily quivering of the lips. Although such quivering may involve both lips, more often, only the lower lip is involved.

Disease causes, disease mechanisms:

I. Stomach fire attacking upward

Stomach fire may be due to contraction of external evils entering the interior and transforming into heat or to addiction to acrid, rich food which gives rise to heat congesting in the stomach. The stomach channel circles the lips. If fire goes up along this channel accompanying externally contracted wind to the lips, there will be tremor in the lips. This is because the nature of wind evils is to move.

2. Blood vacuity & wind dryness

Blood vacuity may be due to enduring disease, contraction of external dry evils, or to improper administration of bitter, cold or warm, dry agents that then damage yin blood. If there is blood vacuity, first, wind is likely to be engendered, and secondly, the sinews and the vessels will lack their proper nourishment. If wind affects the lips and the sinews and vessels associated with the lips lack nourishment, lip tremor will occur.

3. Spleen vacuity not containing

Spleen vacuity may be constitutional or due to dietary irregularities. "The spleen governs the muscles and is associated with the lips." If the spleen becomes vacuous, it may fail to contain and thus the lips will be out of control. Therefore, lip tremor may occur.

Treatment based on pattern discrimination:

I. Stomach fire attacking upward

Symptoms: Lip tremor following red, swollen, itching lips which are burning, painful, and cracked with discharge of watery fluids, dry mouth and thirst, constipation, a red tongue with yellow fur, and a slippery, rapid pulse

Therapeutic principles: Course wind and clear heat

Acupuncture & moxibustion:

Jia Cheng Jiang (M-HN-18) *Cheng Jiang* (CV 24)	Together, these points course wind and clear heat locally.
He Gu (LI 4) *Qu Chi* (LI 11)	Together, these points clear and drain heat in the *yang ming* channel.
Tian Shu (St 25) *Nei Ting* (St 44) *Shang Ju Xu* (St 37)	Together, these points drain heat in the bowels to extinguish wind.

Additions & subtractions: For dizziness, add *Feng Chi* (GB 20).

Chinese medicinal formula: *Fang Feng Tong Sheng San* (Ledebouriella Sagely Unblocking Powder)

Ingredients: Radix Ledebouriellae Divaricatae (*Fang Feng*), 6g, Fructus Forsythiae Suspensae (*Lian Qiao*), 9g, Herba Ephedrae (*Ma Huang*), 3g, Herba Menthae Haplocalysis (*Bo He*), 3g, Herba Schizonepetae Tenuifoliae (*Jing Jie*), 6g, Rhizoma Atractylodis Macrocephalae (*Bai Zhu*), 3g, Fructus Gardeniae Jasminoidis (*Zhi Zi*), 9g, uncooked Radix Ligustici Wallichii (*Chuan Xiong*), 9g, uncooked Radix Angelicae Sinensis (*Dang Gui*), 6g, Radix Albus Paeoniae Lactiflorae (*Bai Shao*), 6g, uncooked Radix Et Rhizoma Rhei (*Da Huang*), 6g, Mirabilitum (*Mang Xiao*), 6g, uncooked Gypsum Fibrosum (*Shi Gao*), 20g, Radix

Scutellariae Baicalensis (*Huang Qin*), 6g, Radix Platycodi Grandiflori (*Jie Geng*), 3g, Radix Glycyrrhizae (*Gan Cao*), 6g, Talcum (*Hua Shi*), 6g

Additions & subtractions: If there is severe constipation, use *Tiao Wei Cheng Qi Tang* (Regulate the Stomach & Order the Qi Decoction): Uncooked Radix Et Rhizoma Rhei (*Da Huang*), 9g, Mirabilitum (*Mang Xiao*), 9g, Radix Glycyrrhizae (*Gan Cao*), 6g.

2. Blood vacuity & wind dryness

Symptoms: Quivering, itchy, dry lips which are often cracked and scaling, vexation, insomnia, uneasy defecation, dry stool, a red tongue with reduced fur, and a fine, rapid pulse

Therapeutic principles: Nourish the blood and dispel wind

Acupuncture & moxibustion:

Cheng Jiang (CV 24)　　Together, these points dispel wind in the lips.
Jia Cheng Jiang (M-HN-18)

Xin Shu (Bl 15)	Together, these points nourish the blood to
Ge Shu (Bl 17)	extinguish wind.
Pi Shu (Bl 20)	
Wei Shu (Bl 21)	

Additions & subtractions: For constipation, add *Shui Dao* (St 28) and *Shang Ju Xu* (St 37).

Chinese medicinal formula: Modified *Si Wu Xiao Feng Yin* (Four Ingredients Disperse Wind Drink)

Ingredients: Uncooked Radix Rehmanniae (*Sheng Di*), 12g, Radix Angelicae Sinensis (*Dang Gui*), 9g, uncooked Radix Albus Paeoniae Lactiflorae (*Bai Shao*), 9g, uncooked Radix Ligustici Wallichii (*Chuan Xiong*), 9g, Cortex Radicis Dictamni Dasycarpi (*Bai Xian Pi*), 6g, Herba

Schizonepetae Tenuifoliae (*Jing Jie*), 6g, Radix Ledebouriellae Divaricatae (*Fang Feng*), 6g, Radix Bupleuri (*Chai Hu*), 6g, Radix Angelicae Pubescentis (*Du Huo*), 6g, Periostracum Cicadae (*Chan Tui*), 15g, Fructus Tribuli Terrestris (*Bai Ji Li*), 6g

3. Spleen vacuity not containing

Symptoms: Tremor of the lips and fingers, reduced food intake, poor appetite, abdominal distention, loose stools, fatigue and lack of strength, a pale, fat, tender tongue with white fur, and a deep, weak, forceless pulse

Therapeutic principles: Supplement the qi and fortify the spleen

Acupuncture & moxibustion:

He Gu (LI 4) *Jia Cheng Jiang* (M-HN-18)	Together, these points free the channels and network vessels.
Qi Hai (CV 6) *Da Du* (Sp 2) *Zu San Li* (St 36)	Together, these points supplement the qi and fortify the spleen (when moxaed on the point of *Da Du*).

Additions & subtractions: For prolapse of the rectum, add *Chang Qiang* (GV 1).

Chinese medicinal formula: Modified *Si Jun Zi Tang* (Four Gentlemen Decoction)

Ingredients: Radix Panacis Ginseng (*Ren Shen*), 6g, Rhizoma Atractylodis Macrocephalae (*Bai Zhu*), 9g, Sclerotium Poriae Cocos (*Fu Ling*), 9g, mix-fried Radix Glycyrrhizae (*Zhi Gan Cao*), 6g, honey stir-fried Radix Astragali Membranacei (*Huang Qi*), 15g, Periostracum Cicadae (*Chan Tui*), 15g

18
Swelling, Itching & Pain in the Lips
(*Chun Zhong Yang Tong*)

This disease category refers to red, swollen lips that are itching and painful.

Disease causes, disease mechanisms:

Heat accumulation in the stomach

This heat may be from contraction of external evils entering the interior and then transforming into heat and then accumulating in the stomach or from addiction to acrid, rich food which engenders heat. The stomach channel encircles the lips. If accumulated heat goes upward to the lips along this channel, there will be swollen, itchy, painful lips.

Treatment based on pattern discrimination:

Heat accumulation in the stomach

Symptoms: Red, swollen, itchy, painful lips, thirst with desire for chilled drinks, constipation, a red tongue with yellow fur, and a rapid pulse

Therapeutic principles: Clear heat and drain fire

Acupuncture & moxibustion:

Ren Zhong (GV 26)   Together, these points clear heat in the local area.
Cheng Jiang (CV 26)

He Gu (LI 4)	Together, these points clear heat and drain fire in
Qu Chi (LI 11)	the *yang ming*.
San Jian (LI 3)	
Jie Xi (St 41)	

Additions & subtractions: For bad breath, add *Da Ling* (Per 7). For toothache, add *Jiao Sun* (TB 20).

Chinese medicinal formula: *Tiao Wei Cheng Qi Tang* (Regulate the Stomach & Order the Qi Decoction)

Ingredients: Uncooked Radix Et Rhizoma Rhei (*Da Huang*), 9g, Mirabilitum (*Mang Xiao*), 9g, Radix Glycyrrhizae (*Gan Cao*), 6g

Additions & subtractions: If redness, swelling, itching, and pain of the lips are severe but without severe constipation, use *Bai Hu Tang* (White Tiger Decoction): Uncooked Gypsum Fibrosum (*Shi Gao*), 30g, uncooked Rhizoma Anemarrhenae Asphodeloidis (*Zhi Mu*), 9g, Radix Glycyrrhizae (*Gan Cao*), 6g, Semen Oryzae Sativae (*Geng Mi*), 9g. If constipation is severe, increase the dosage of Radix Et Rhizoma Rhei (*Da Huang*) and Mirabilitum (*Mang Xiao*). For lingering swollen, itchy, painful lips, use *Yi Yi Ren Tang* (Coicis Decoction): Semen Coicis Lachryma-jobi (*Yi Yi Ren*), 20g, Semen Phaseoli Calcarati (*Chi Xiao Dou*), 12g, Radix Stephaniae Tetrandrae (*Han Fang Ji*), 9g, Radix Glycyrrhizae (*Gan Cao*), 6g

19
Swollen Tongue (*She Zhong*)

Swollen tongue refers to enlargement of the tongue which may also possibly be hard and painful. The tongue may be so swollen as to jam the mouth and thus affect eating, speaking, and breathing.

Disease causes, disease mechanisms:

I. Contraction of external wind cold

Wind evils are mobile and cold evils are congealing. The heart opens into the tongue, while the spleen channel connects with the root of the tongue. If wind cold attacks the body, entering the heart and spleen channels, the wind may draft the cold upward to the tongue. This then results in congelation of the blood and blockage of the vessels therein. Therefore, the tongue will be swollen.

2. Depressed fire in the heart channel

Essence spirit (*i.e.*, mental-emotional) dissatisfaction or over-thinking may lead to depression of the five affects which, over time, may transform fire. If this fire renders heart fire extremely exuberant, exuberant heart fire will harass the tongue along its channel, burning the network vessels and causing blockage therein. Thus swollen tongue will occur.

3. Heat accumulation in the heart & spleen

This accumulation of heat may be due to constitutional phlegm heat exuberance in the interior and/or from the addiction to alcohol. If this accumulated heat produces toxins over time and goes upward to and congeals in the tongue, there will be a swollen tongue.

4. Spleen vacuity

Spleen vacuity may be constitutional or may be due to dietary irregularities and enduring disease which damages spleen yang. If there is spleen vacuity, dampness will engender and collect in the interior. If water dampness goes upward along the spleen channel to the tongue and congeals and blocks the qi mechanism there, swollen tongue will occur.

Treatment based on pattern discrimination:

I. Contraction of external wind cold

Symptoms: Sudden onset of tongue pain, hardness, and swelling, a dark purple tongue which is not red in color, aversion to cold, fever, body aches, a bland taste in the mouth, no thought for food, chilly pain in the abdomen, diarrhea, heart palpitations, blurred speech, and a floating, tight pulse

Therapeutic principles: Course and dissipate evils in the heart and spleen

Acupuncture & moxibustion:

Lian Quan (CV 23) *Jin Jin Yu Ye* (M-HN-20)	Together, these points unblock the network vessels.
Shao Shang (Lu 11) *Shang Yang* (LI 1) *He Gu* (LI 4) *Wai Guan* (TB 5)	Together, these points course wind and dissipate cold.

Chinese medicinal formula: *Jin Fo Cao San* (Inula Powder)

Ingredients: Flos Inulae (*Xuan Fu Hua*), 9g, uncooked Herba Ephedrae (*Ma Huang*), 9g, Radix Peucedani (*Qian Hu*), 9g, Herba Schizonepetae Tenuifoliae (*Jing Jie*), 9g, ginger stir-fried Rhizoma Pinelliae Ternatae (*Ban Xia*), 6g, Radix Rubrus Paeoniae Lactiflorae (*Chi Shao*), 6g, Radix Glycyrrhizae (*Gan Cao*), 3g, uncooked Rhizoma Zingiberis (*Sheng Jiang*), 6g, Fructus Zizyphi Jujubae (*Da Zao*), 3 fruits

2. Depressed fire in the heart channel

Symptoms: Sudden onset of a red, painful, swollen tongue which, in severe cases, can jam the mouth, thus affecting eating and speaking, a red face, vexation and agitation, restlessness, short voidings of yellow urine, a bitter taste in the mouth, and a rapid pulse which is surging and big at the *cun* on the left side.

Therapeutic principles: Clear the heart and drain fire

Acupuncture & moxibustion:

Shi Xuan (M-UE-1)   Together, these points clear the heart and drain
Hai Quan (M-HN-37)   fire when pricked to bleed.
Jin Jin Yu Ye (M-HN-20)

Chinese medicinal formula: Modified *Qing Xin Liang Ge San* (Clear the Heart & Cool the Diaphragm Powder)

Ingredients: Fructus Forsythiae Suspensae (*Lian Qiao*), 9g, uncooked Rhizoma Coptidis Chinensis (*Huang Lian*), 9g, Fructus Gardeniae Jasminoidis (*Zhi Zi*), 9g, Herba Menthae Haplocalysis (*Bo He*), 3g, uncooked Gypsum Fibrosum (*Shi Gao*), 20g, Folium Bambusae (*Zhu Ye*), 12g, Radix Platycodi Grandiflori (*Jie Geng*), 3g, Radix Glycyrrhizae (*Gan Cao*), 6g

3. Heat accumulation in the heart & spleen

Symptoms: A red, swollen tongue which may jam the mouth, anxiety and agitation, burning heat in the palms and skin, preference for a cold environment, thirst with no desire to drink, lassitude with no willingness to move, short voidings of dark-colored urine, constipation, possibly full, yellow, and glossy tongue fur, and a slippery, rapid pulse

Therapeutic principles: Clear heat and drain fire, resolve toxins and transform dampness

Acupuncture & moxibustion:

Shen Men (Ht 7) *Da Ling* (Per 7)	Together, these points drain fire and resolve toxins.
Yin Bai (Sp 1) *San Yin Jiao* (Sp 6) *Yin Ling Quan* (Sp 9)	Together, these points clear and eliminate dampness and heat.

Additions & subtractions: For inhibited defecation, add *Tian Shu* (St 25).

Chinese medicinal formula: *Xie Huang San* (Drain the Yellow Powder) plus *Zhi Zi Da Huang Tang* (Gardenia & Rhubarb Decoction)

Ingredients: Radix Ledebouriellae Divaricatae (*Fang Feng*), 6g, Fructus Gardeniae Jasminoidis (*Zhi Zi*), 9g, Herba Agastachis Seu Pogostemi (*Huo Xiang*), 6g, Gypsum Fibrosum (*Shi Gao*), 15g, Radix Glycyrrhizae (*Gan Cao*), 6g, uncooked Radix Et Rhizoma Rhei (*Da Huang*), 9g, Fructus Immaturus Citri Aurantii (*Zhi Shi*), 6g, Semen Praeparatus Sojae (*Dan Dou Chi*), 6g

4. Spleen vacuity

Symptoms: A dull, pale, swollen tongue with teeth-prints on its edges and watery, glossy fur, a pale yellow facial complexion, encumbered limbs, lassitude and lack of strength, abdominal distention and fullness which is worse after eating, no desire to drink, long voidings of clear urine, loose stools, and a deep, moderate (*i.e.*, relaxed) pulse

Therapeutic principles: Supplement qi and fortify the spleen, warm and move center yang

Acupuncture & moxibustion:

Lian Quan (CV 23)	Frees the flow of the network vessels in the local area
Zhong Wan (CV 12) *Jian Li* (CV 11) *Zu San Li* (St 37) *Gong Sun* (Sp 4)	Together, these points fortify the spleen and regulate the stomach.

Additions & subtractions: For dizziness, add *Bai Hui* (GV 20).

Chinese medicinal formula: *Shen Ling Bai Zhu San* (Ginseng, Poria & Atractylodes Powder)

Ingredients: Stir-fried Semen Dolichoris Lablab (*Bai Bian Dou*), 9g, stir-fried Radix Dioscoreae Oppositae (*Shan Yao*), 9g, bran stir-fried Rhizoma Atractylodis Macrocephalae (*Bai Zhu*), 9g, Sclerotium Poriae Cocos (*Fu Ling*), 9g, rice stir-fried Radix Codonopsitis Pilosulae (*Dang Shen*), 9g, stir-fried till yellow Semen Nelumbinis Nuciferae (*Lian Zi*), 9g, Radix Platycodi Grandiflori (*Jie Geng*), 3g, Semen Coicis Lachryma-jobi (*Yi Yi Ren*), 15g, Fructus Amomi (*Sha Ren*), 6g, mix-fried Radix Glycyrrhizae (*Zhi Gan Cao*), 3g

Additions & subtractions: If spleen yang vacuity is predominant, subtract Semen Dolichoris Lablab (*Bai Bian Dou*), Semen Coicis Lachryma-jobi (*Yi Yi Ren*), and Radix Platycodi Grandiflori (*Jie Geng*) and add bland Radix Lateralis Praeparatus Aconiti Carmichaeli (*Fu Zi*), 6g, and dry Rhizoma Zingiberis (*Gan Jiang*), 6g.

20
Fat Tongue (*She Pang*)

This refers to a puffy, enlarged tongue with possible teeth-prints on its edges. However, in this case, the tongue is not nearly as swollen and enlarged as in swollen tongue above. In the above case, the tongue is so swollen as to affect eating, speaking, and even possibly breathing. Here, the patient has no subjective sensation of their tongue being puffy and enlarged. This condition is only diagnosed by visual inspection when the patient is asked to stick out their tongue.

Disease causes, disease mechanisms:

I. Spleen yang vacuity

Spleen yang vacuity may be constitutional or due to dietary irregularities or enduring disease. It may also develop from spleen qi vacuity, kidney yang vacuity, or failure of fire to engender earth. With spleen yang vacuity, water dampness and yin cold will collect in the interior. If yin cold counterflows upward and spills over into the tongue, a fat tongue will occur.

2. Kidney yang vacuity

Kidney yang vacuity may be constitutional or due to aging, enduring disease, or sexual taxation. If there is kidney yang vacuity, there will be failure of qi transformation leading to yin cold exuberance in the interior. If this yin cold spills over into the tongue above, a fat tongue will occur.

Treatment based on pattern discrimination:

I. Spleen yang vacuity

Symptoms: A pale, tender, fat tongue with teeth-prints on its edges and rich liquids on its surface accompanied by a withered white facial complexion, cold form (*i.e.*, body) and chilled limbs, a low voice while speaking, fatigue and lack of strength, reduced food intake, loose stools, white and glossy or slimy tongue fur, and a fine, soft, or deep, moderate (*i.e.*, relaxed) pulse

Therapeutic principles: Boost the qi with sweet, warm medicinals, warm yang and dissipate cold

Acupuncture & moxibustion:

Lian Quan (CV 23)	Together, these points disinhibit dampness and
Dui Duan (GV 27)	dissipate cold in the local area.

Qi Hai (CV 6)	Together, when moxaed, these points boost the qi
Guan Yuan (CV 4)	and fortify the spleen to disinhibit the dampness.
Da Du (Sp 2)	
Zu San Li (St 36)	

Additions & subtractions: For insomnia at night but somnolence during the daytime, add *Shen Mai* (Bl 62) and *Zhao Hai* (Ki 6).

Chinese medicinal formula: Modified *Liu Jun Zi Tang* (Six Gentlemen Decoction)

Ingredients: Rice stir-fried Radix Codonopsitis Pilosulae (*Dang Shen*), 9g, bran stir-fried Rhizoma Atractylodis Macrocephalae (*Bai Zhu*), 6g, Sclerotium Poriae Cocos (*Fu Ling*), 6g, mix-fried Radix Glycyrrhizae (*Zhi Gan Cao*), 3g, uncooked Rhizoma Zingiberis (*Sheng Jiang*), 6g, stir-fried

Pericarpium Citri Reticulatae (*Chen Pi*), 6g, lime-processed Rhizoma Pinelliae Ternatae (*Ban Xia*), 6g, dry Rhizoma Zingiberis (*Gan Jiang*), 6g, bland Radix Lateralis Praeparatus Aconiti Carmichaeli (*Fu Zi*), 6g

2. Kidney yang vacuity

Symptoms: A pale, tender, fat tongue with teeth-prints on its tip and edges and profuse drool in the mouth accompanied by counterflow chilling of the limbs, cold form, a curled-up lying posture, lassitude of the spirit, edema especially below the waist, inhibited defecation, and a deep, slow pulse

Therapeutic principles: Warm yang and dissipate cold, disinhibit water and disperse swelling

Acupuncture & moxibustion:

Lian Quan (CV 23)   Together, these points disinhibit water in the local
Hai Quan (M-HN-37)   area.

Qi Hai (CV 6)   Together, when moxaed, these points warm yang
Guan Yuan (CV 4)   and dissipate cold to disinhibit the water.
Ming Men (GV 4)

Yin Ling Quan (Sp 9)   Disperses swelling

Chinese medicinal formula: Modified *Zhen Wu Tang* (True Warrior Decoction)

Ingredients: Bland Radix Lateralis Praeparatus Aconiti Carmichaeli (*Fu Zi*), 6g, uncooked Rhizoma Atractylodis Macrocephalae (*Bai Zhu*), 9g, Radix Albus Paeoniae Lactiflorae (*Bai Shao*), 6g, uncooked Rhizoma Zingiberis (*Sheng Jiang*), 9g, Sclerotium Poriae Cocos (*Fu Ling*), 9g, Semen Plantaginis (*Che Qian Zi*), 6g, stir-fried Ramulus Cinnamomi

Cassiae (*Gui Zhi*), 9g, prepared Radix Rehmanniae (*Shu Di*), 18g, salt mix-fried Rhizoma Alismatis (*Ze Xie*), 9g

21
Trembling Tongue (*She Chan*)

Trembling tongue refers to involuntary shaking of the tongue, especially when the patient is asked to stick out their tongue.

Disease causes, disease mechanisms:

I. Qi and blood vacuity

Qi and blood vacuity may be due to constitutional insufficiency, spleen-stomach vacuity, chronic or massive bleeding, enduring disease, or over-thinking. If the qi and blood become vacuous, they may not nourish the sinews properly, thus leading to tremor. If the sinews of the tongue are affected, trembling of the tongue will occur.

2. Liver wind stirring internally

Liver wind may stir internally if a) there is extreme heat from external evils or excesses of the five affects that burn the liver channel, b) there is liver-kidney yin vacuity from aging, unrestrained sexual activity, or enduring disease leaving liver yang unchecked, or c) there is yin vacuity from yin humors consumption by warm evils lingering in the body during the late stage of a warm disease or due to enduring disease. "The liver governs the sinews" and "Wind is mobile by nature." If liver wind stirs internally, tremors will occur, leading to trembling of the tongue.

3. Alcohol toxins brewing internally

Alcohol can easily enter the channels and network vessels and engender heat, burning and consuming yin humors. Thus an enduring addiction to alcohol may result in alcohol toxins brewing internally and less nourishment and moistening for the sinews. Therefore, trembling of the tongue may occur.

Treatment based on pattern discrimination:

I. Qi and blood vacuity

Symptoms: Trembling of the tongue when the tongue is stuck out accompanied by heart palpitations, racing heart, insomnia, sleep with profuse dreaming, impaired memory it, lack of strength, fatigue, dizziness, flowery (*i.e.*, blurred) vision, a lusterless facial complexion, tingling and numbness in the hands and feet, possible scanty menstruation in women, a pale red tongue, and a fine, forceless pulse

Therapeutic principles: Nourish the blood and moisten the sinews, supplement and boost the heart and spleen

Acupuncture & moxibustion:

Lian Quan (CV 23)   Moistens the sinews of the tongue

Xin Shu (Bl 15)   Together, these points nourish the blood and
Ge Shu (Bl 17)   supplement and boost the heart and spleen.
Pi Shu (Bl 20)
Wei Shu (Bl 21)

Additions: For menstrual problems in women, add *San Yin Jiao* (Sp 6).

Chinese medicinal formula: Modified *Ba Zhen Tang* (Eight Pearls Decoction)

Ingredients: Prepared Radix Rehmanniae (*Shu Di*), 12g, Radix Angelicae Sinensis (*Dang Gui*), 9g, Radix Albus Paeoniae Lactiflorae (*Bai Shao*), 15g, uncooked Radix Ligustici Wallichii (*Chuan Xiong*), 6g, honey stir-fried Radix Codonopsitis Pilosulae (*Dang Shen*), 9g, bran stir-fried Rhizoma Atractylodis Macrocephalae (*Bai Zhu*), 9g, Sclerotium Poriae Cocos (*Fu Ling*), 9g, mix-fried Radix Glycyrrhizae (*Zhi Gan Cao*), 6g, Fructus Chaenomlis Lagenariae (*Mu Gua*), 9g

Additions & subtractions: If qi vacuity is predominant, use Modified *Gui Pi Tang* (Return the Spleen Decoction): Bran stir-fried Rhizoma Atractylodis Macrocephalae (*Bai Zhu*), 9g, Sclerotium Poriae Cocos (*Fu Ling*), 9g, honey mix-fried Radix Astragali Membranacei (*Huang Qi*), 15g, rice stir-fried Radix Codonopsitis Pilosulae (*Dang Shen*), 9g, mix-fried Radix Glycyrrhizae (*Zhu Gan Cao*), 6g, wine-processed Radix Angelicae Sinensis (*Dang Gui*), 6g, uncooked Radix Albus Paeoniae Lactiflorae (*Bai Shao*), 9g, stir-fried Semen Zizyphi Spinosae (*Suan Zao Ren*), 6g.

2. Extreme heat engendering wind

Symptoms: Trembling of the tongue accompanied by fever, vexation and agitation, dizziness, distention and pain in the head, convulsions, clouded spirit in severe cases, a crimson tongue, and a wiry, rapid pulse

Therapeutic principles: Cool the liver and extinguish wind

Acupuncture & moxibustion:

Jin Jin Yu Ye (M-HN-20)   Together, these points drain heat.
Shi Xuan (M-UE-1)

Tai Chong (Liv 3)   Together, these points cool the liver and
Xia Xi (GB 43)   extinguish wind.
Yong Quan (Ki 1)

Additions & subtractions: For clouded spirit, add *Ren Zhong* (GV 26).

Chinese medicinal formula: Modified *Ling Yang Jiao Gou Teng Tang* (Antelope Horn & Gastrodia Decoction)

Ingredients: Cornu Caprae (*Shan Yang Jiao*), 15g, Ramulus Uncariae Cum Uncis (*Gou Teng*), 12g, Caulis Bambusae In Taeniis (*Zhu Ru*), 6g, uncooked Radix Rehmanniae (*Sheng Di*), 15g, Folium Mori Albi (*Sang Ye*), 9g, Bulbus Fritillariae Thunbergii (*Zhe Bei Mu*), 6g, Flos Chrysanthemi Morifolii (*Ju Hua*), 15g, Sclerotium Pararadicis Poriae Cocos (*Fu Shen*), 9g, Radix Albus Paeoniae Lactiflorae (*Bai Shao*), 12g, Radix Glycyrrhizae (*Gan Cao*), 3g

Note: Since Saiga antelope horn is from an endangered species, we have substituted goat horn (Cornu Caprae, *Shan Yang Jiao*) in all standard formulas containing Saiga antelope horn.

3. Liver yang transforming wind

Symptoms: Trembling tongue accompanied by trembling and hypertonic limbs, vertigo, agitation, possible insomnia, sleep with profuse dreaming, unsteady steps, clouding collapse and deviation of the mouth and eyes in severe cases, a red tongue, and a wiry, forceful pulse

Therapeutic principles: Level the liver, subdue yang, and extinguish wind

Acupuncture & moxibustion:

Lian Quan (CV 23)	Harmonizes the network vessels
Tai Chong (Liv 3) *Xing Jian* (Liv 2)	Together, these points level the liver.
Tai Xi (Ki 3) *San Yin Jiao* (Sp 6)	Together, these points enrich yin to subdue yang and extinguish wind.

Chinese medicinal formula: *Zhen Gan Xi Feng Tang* (Settle the Liver & Extinguish Wind Decoction)

Ingredients: Uncooked Os Draconis (*Long Gu*), 15g, uncooked Concha Ostreae (*Mu Li*), 15g, uncooked Haemititum (*Dai Zhe Shi*), 15g, salt stir-fried Radix Achyranthis Bidentatae (*Niu Xi*), 15g, uncooked Plastrum Testudinis (*Gui Ban*), 15g, Radix Scrophulariae Ningpoensis (*Xuan Shen*), 6g, Tuber Asparagi Cochinensis (*Tian Men Dong*), 6g, uncooked Radix Albus Paeoniae Lactiflorae (*Bai Shao*), 15g, Herba Artemisiae Capillaris (*Yin Chen Hao*), 6g, Fructus Meliae Toosendan (*Chuan Lian Zi*), 6g, Fructus Germinatus Hordei Vulgaris (*Mai Ya*), 6g, Radix Glycyrrhizae (*Gan Cao*), 6g

4. Yin vacuity & wind stirring

Symptoms: Slight trembling of the tongue accompanied by fever which is worse at night, fatigue, deafness, trembling limbs, a crimson tongue with peeled fur, and a vacuous, weak pulse

Therapeutic principles: Enrich yin and extinguish wind

Acupuncture & moxibustion:

Lian Quan (CV 23)	Harmonizes the network vessels
Tai Xi (Ki 3)	Together, these points enrich yin, clear heat,
Fu Liu (Ki 7)	and extinguish wind.
San Yin Jiao (Sp 6)	

Additions & subtractions: For insomnia, add *Feng Chi* (GB 20) and *An Mian* (N-BW-21).

Chinese medicinal formula: *San Jia Fu Mai Tang* (Three Shells Restore the Pulse Decoction)

Ingredients: Uncooked Concha Ostreae (*Mu Li*), 15g, uncooked Plastrum Testudinis (*Gui Ban*), 15g, uncooked Carapax Amydae Sinensis (*Bie Jia*), 15g, uncooked Radix Rehmanniae (*Sheng Di*), 15g, uncooked Radix Albus Paeoniae Lactiflorae (*Bai Shao*), 15g, Tuber Ophiopogonis Japonici (*Mai Men Dong*), 6g, Gelatinum Corii Asini (*E Jiao*), 6g, Semen Cannabis Sativae (*Huo Ma Ren*), 6g, Radix Glycyrrhizae (*Gan Cao*), 3g

5. Alcohol toxins brewing internally

Symptoms: A fat, trembling tongue, thirst, profuse phlegm, trembling limbs, a history of alcohol addiction, a purple-red tongue with thick fur, and a rapid pulse

Therapeutic principles: Clear and resolve alcohol toxins

Acupuncture & moxibustion:

Lian Quan (CV 23)	Harmonizes the network vessels
Gong Sun (Sp 4)	Together, these points fortify the spleen, disinhibit
Dan Shu (Bl 19)	dampness, and resolve toxins.
Zhi Yang (GV 9)	
Wei Zhong (Bl 40)	
Hand Wan Gu (SI 4)	

Chinese medicinal formula: Modified *Ge Hua Jie Cheng Tang* (Pueraria Flower Resolve Alcoholism Decoction)

Ingredients: Flos Puerariae (*Ge Hua*), 9g, Fructus Cardamomi (*Bai Dou Kou*), 9g, Fructus Amomi (*Sha Ren*), 6g, Radix Auklandiae Lappae (*Mu Xiang*), 9g, Pericarpium Citri Reticulatae (*Chen Pi*), 9g, Pericarpium Citri Reticulatae Viride (*Qing Pi*), 6g, Radix Codonopsitis Pilosulae (*Dang Shen*), 6g, Rhizoma Atractylodis Macrocephalae (*Bai Zhu*), 9g, Sclerotium Poriae Cocos (*Fu Ling*), 9g, stir-fried Massa Medica Fermentata (*Shen Qu*), 9g, dry Rhizoma Zingiberis (*Gan Jiang*), 3g,

Sclerotium Polypori Umbellati (*Zhu Ling*), 6g, Rhizoma Alismatis (*Ze Xie*), 6g, stir-fried Fructus Crataegi (*Shan Zha*), 9g

22
Stiff Tongue (*She Qiang*)

Stiff tongue refers to the patient's inability to move their tongue agilely. Thus, their speech is also inhibited.

Disease causes, disease mechanisms:

I. Wind phlegm obstruction

This wind mainly comes from liver-kidney yin vacuity rendering yang unchecked or from excesses of the five affects transforming into fire and then engendering wind. The phlegm may be constitutional or may be due to dietary irregularities that damage the spleen. Thus the spleen fails to transform dampness and this dampness accumulates and eventually is congealed into phlegm. It is also possible for heat to burn liquids into phlegm. If wind drafts this phlegm upward resulting in blockage of the root of the tongue or clouds the clear portals, there will be stiff tongue. Stiff tongue due to wind phlegm obstruction is usually associated with the sequelae of windstroke or apoplexy.

2. Heat blocking the portals of the heart

In warm disease, warm heat evils may fall inward to the pericardium due to faulty practice or delayed treatment or if warm heat evils are extremely strong while there is heart yin vacuity. The tongue is the portal of the heart. If heat blocks the heart portal, the spirit brightness will be in chaos and hence the tongue will lose its agility, thus becoming stiff.

Treatment based on pattern discrimination:

I. Wind phlegm blocking the network vessels

Symptoms: Stiff tongue with inhibited speech possibly accompanied by deviated mouth and eyes and/or hemiplegia. In some cases, there may be a deviated tongue which is difficult to stretch out. In addition, there is slimy, thick tongue fur, and a floating, wiry or floating, slippery pulse.

Therapeutic principles: Dispel wind, transform phlegm, and unblock the network vessels

Acupuncture & moxibustion:

Lian Quan (CV 23)   Together, these points unblock the network vessels
Cheng Jiang (CV 24)   and disinhibit the portal.

Guan Chong (TB 1)   Together, these points dispel wind.
Hand *Zhong Zhu* (TB 3)
Wai Guan (TB 5)

Additions & subtractions: Add *Feng Long* (St 40) when there are obvious signs of phlegm.

Chinese medicinal formula: Modified *Qian Zheng San* (Lead to Symmetry Powder)

Ingredients: Uncooked Rhizoma Typhonii Gigantei (*Bai Fu Zi*), 9g, uncooked Bombyx Batryticatus (*Jiang Can*), 6g, Buthus Martensi (*Quan Xie*), 6g, lime-processed Rhizoma Pinelliae Ternatae (*Ban Xia*), 9g, uncooked Rhizoma Atractylodis Macrocephalae (*Bai Zhu*), 9g, stir-fried till yellow Rhizoma Gastrodiae Elatae (*Tian Ma*), 9g, Pericarpium Citri Reticulatae (*Chen Pi*), 6g, Sclerotium Poriae Cocos (*Fu Ling*), 6g, Rhizoma Arisaematis (*Tian Nan Xing*), 6g, Radix Glycyrrhizae (*Gan Cao*), 3g

Additions & subtractions: If there is only external wind network vessel stroke (*wai feng zhong luo*), use *Da Qin Jiao Tang* (Major Gentiana Macrophylla Decoction): Radix Gentianae Macrophyllae (*Qin Jiao*), 9g, uncooked Radix Ligustici Wallichii (*Chuan Xiong*), 9g, Radix Angelicae Sinensis (*Dang Gui*), 6g, Radix Albus Paeoniae Lactiflorae (*Bai Shao*), 6g, Herba Asari Cum Radice (*Xi Xin*), 3g, Radix Et Rhizoma Notopterygii (*Qiang Huo*), 6g, Radix Ledebouriellae Divaricatae (*Fang Feng*), 6g, Radix Scutellariae Baicalensis (*Huang Qin*), 6g, uncooked Gypsum Fibrosum (*Shi Gao*), 12g, Radix Angelicae Dahuricae (*Bai Zhi*), 3g, Rhizoma Atractylodis Macrocephalae (*Bai Zhu*), 6g, uncooked Radix Rehmanniae (*Sheng Di*), 6g, prepared Radix Rehmanniae (*Shu Di*), 6g, Sclerotium Poriae Cocos (*Fu Ling*), 6g, Radix Angelicae Pubescentis (*Du Huo*), 6g, Radix Glycyrrhizae (*Gan Cao*), 6g

2. Liver wind stirring internally

Symptoms: Sudden clouding collapse followed by coma, clenched jaw, phlegm rales in the throat, a stiff tongue which is difficult to stretch out for inspection, slimy tongue fur, and a wiry, rapid, slippery pulse

Therapeutic principles: Sweep away the phlegm, extinguish the wind, and open the portals

Acupuncture & moxibustion:

Lian Quan (CV 23) *Ren Zhong* (GV 26)	Together, these points unblock the network vessels and disinhibit the portals.
Feng Long (St 40) *Nei Ting* (St 44)	Together, these points transform phlegm and clear heat.
Tai Chong (Liv 3) *Yong Quan* (Ki 1)	Together, these points clear heat, extinguish wind, and open the portals.

Additions & subtractions: For deviated mouth and eye, add *Zan Zhu* (Bl 2), *Yang Bai* (GB 14), *Di Cang* (St 4), *He Gu* (LI 4) and *Jia Che* (St 6). For hemiplegia, add *Ji Quan* (Ht 1), *Chi Ze* (Lu 5), *He Gu* (LI 4), *Ba Xie* (M-UE-22), *Jian Yu* (LI 15), *Qu Chi* (LI 11), *Wai Guan* (TB 5), *San Yin Jiao* (Sp 6), *Wei Zhong* (Bl 40), *Yang Ling Quan* (GB 34), *Jie Xi* (St 41), and *Qiu Xu* (GB 40).

Chinese medicinal formula: Modified *Di Tan Tang* (Flush Phlegm Decoction)

Ingredients: Lime-processed Rhizoma Pinelliae Ternatae (*Ban Xia*), 9g, bile-processed Rhizoma Arisaematis (*Dan Nan Xing*), 9g, Pericarpium Citri Reticulatae (*Chen Pi*), 6g, Fructus Immaturus Citri Aurantii (*Zhi Shi*), 6g, Sclerotium Poriae Cocos (*Fu Ling*), 9g, Radix Codonopsitis Pilosulae (*Dang Shen*), 6g, Caulis Bambusae In Taeniis (*Zhu Ru*), 6g, Rhizoma Acori Graminei (*Shi Chang Pu*), 9g, Styrax Liquidus (*Su He Xiang*), 1g (powder and take with the strained decoction; do not cook), Borneol (*Bing Pian*), 0.5g (powder and take with the strained decoction; do not cook), uncooked Rhizoma Zingiberis (*Sheng Jiang*), 3g, Radix Glycyrrhizae (*Gan Cao*), 3g

3. Phlegm confounding the portals of the heart

Symptoms: Sudden clouding collapse, coma, stiff tongue, foamy drooling, convulsions, and then spontaneous restoration of consciousness, white, slimy tongue fur, and a slippery pulse

Therapeutic principles: Sweep away the phlegm and extinguish the wind

Acupuncture & moxibustion:

Ren Zhong (GV 26)   Arouses the spirit, opens the portals, and settles tetany

Nei Guan (Per 6)	Together, these points rectify the qi, transform
Zu San Li (St 36)	phlegm, and extinguish wind.
Feng Long (St 40)	
Feng Chi (GB 20)	

Chinese medicinal formula: Modified *Ding Xian Wan* (Stabilize Seizure Pills)

Ingredients: Stir-fried till yellow Rhizoma Gastrodiae Elatae (*Tian Ma*), 12g, Bulbus Fritillariae Cirrhosae (*Chuan Bei Mu*), 6g, lime-processed Rhizoma Pinelliae Ternatae (*Ban Xia*), 9g, Sclerotium Poriae Cocos (*Fu Ling*), 9g, Sclerotium Pararadicis Poriae Cocos (*Fu Shen*), 9g, bile-processed Rhizoma Arisaematis (*Dan Nan Xing*), 9g, Rhizoma Acori Graminei (*Shi Chang Pu*), 6g, Radix Glycyrrhizae (*Gan Cao*), 3g, uncooked Bombyx Batryticatus (*Jiang Can*), 9g, Succinum (*Hu Po*), 1g, (powder and take with the strained decoction), Pericarpium Citri Reticulatae (*Chen Pi*), 6g, licorice-processed Radix Polygalae Tenuifoliae (*Yuan Zhi*), 6g, Radix Salviae Miltiorrhizae (*Dan Shen*), 9g, Buthus Martensi (*Quan Xie*), 3g, Concretio Silicea Bambusae (*Tian Zhu Huang*), 9g

4. Heat blocking the portals of the heart

Symptoms: A stiff, crimson tongue, counterflow chilling of the limbs, high fever, coma, clouding with no speech or delirium, and a surging, large, rapid pulse

Therapeutic principles: Clear the heart and open the portals

Acupuncture and moxibustion:

Lian Quan (CV 23)	Unblocks the network vessels and disinhibits the portals

Shi Xuan (M-UE-1)   Clears the heart, opens the portals, and arouses the spirit

Additions & subtractions: For yellow tongue fur which suggests heat bind in the bowels and that this heat has fallen inward to the pericardium, add *Nei Ting* (St 44) and *Yong Quan* (Ki 1). Add *Ran Gu* (Ki 2) and *Fu Liu* (Ki 7) when there is persistent tidal fever and vexation implying that yin humors are exhausted.

Chinese medicinal formula: Modified *An Gong Niu Huang Wan* (Quiet the Palace Bezoar Pills)

Ingredients: Calculus Bovis (*Niu Huang*), 0.5g (not decocted), Tuber Curcumae (*Yu Jin*), 9g, Cornu Bubali (*Shui Niu Jiao*), 30g, Rhizoma Coptidis Chinensis (*Huang Lian*), 9g, Cinnabar (*Zhu Sha*), 0.5g (not decocted), Borneol (*Bing Pian*), 0.5g (not decocted), Secretio Moschi Moschiferi (*She Xiang*), 0.05 (not decocted), Margarita (*Zhen Zhu*), 0.5g (powdered), Fructus Gardeniae Jasminoidis (*Zhi Zi*), 9g, Realgar (*Xiong Huang*), 0.5g (not decocted), Radix Scutellariae Baicalensis (*Huang Qin*), 9g

Decoct the Curcuma, water buffalo horn, Coptis, Scutellaria, and Gardenia first. Then take the other ingredients washed down with the warm decoction. The above dosage is for one day.

23
Numbness of the Tongue (*She Ma*)

Numbness of the tongue refers to an inability to feel the tongue accompanied by a possible tingling sensation.

Disease causes, disease mechanisms:

I. Blood vacuity

Blood vacuity may be due to massive loss of blood, chronic bleeding, congenital spleen-stomach vacuity, dietary irregularities that damage the spleen, or over-thinking that insidiously consumes the heart blood. "Blood vacuity leads to numbness." If the blood is vacuous and fails to nourish the tongue, there will be tongue numbness.

2. Liver wind stirring internally

Aging, enduring disease, or sexual taxation can lead to liver-kidney yin vacuity. Yin is supposed to check yang. Being vacuous, liver-kidney yin cannot check liver yang properly. In that case, unchecked liver yang will become hyperactive and transform into wind which flows upward and harasses the clear portals. This then results in numbness of the tongue.

3. Phlegm blockage

Phlegm can be constitutional or from dietary irregularities that damage the spleen, leading to the accumulation of dampness and thus eventually phlegm. If there is a contraction of the external wind or heat or there is internal heat from enduring phlegm accumulation or from excesses of the five affects, such wind or heat may take the phlegm upward to block the network vessels or channels that connect with the tongue. If these become blocked, the qi mechanism will be inhibited and, therefore, there will be less nourishment to the sinews and network vessels of the tongue. Thus, numbness of the tongue may occur.

Treatment based on pattern discrimination:

I. Blood vacuity

Symptoms: A numb, pale tongue with no hypertonicity, a lusterless facial complexion, heart palpitations, qi shortage, fatigue and lack of strength, insomnia, impaired memory, and a fine, weak pulse

Therapeutic principles: Supplement and nourish the blood

Acupuncture & moxibustion:

Tong Li (Ht 5)	Together, these points supplement and boost the
Lian Quan (CV 23)	network vessels when needled with supplementing method.

San Yin Jiao (Sp 6)	Together, these points supplement the blood.
Zu San Li (St 36)	

Chinese medicinal formula: Modified *Si Wu Tang* (Four Ingredients Decoction)

Ingredients: Prepared Radix Rehmanniae (*Shu Di*), 12g, uncooked Radix Albus Paeoniae Lactiflorae (*Bai Shao*), 12g, wine mix-fried Radix Angelicae Sinensis (*Dang Gui*), 9g, wine mix-fried Radix Ligustici Wallichii (*Chuan Xiong*), 6g, Gelatinum Corii Asini (*E Jiao*), 12g, Arillus Euphoriae Longanae (*Long Yan Rou*), 9g, uncooked Radix Codonopsitis Pilosulae (*Dang Shen*), 9g, wine mix-fried Radix Salviae Miltiorrhizae (*Dan Shen*), 9g, mix-fried Radix Glycyrrhizae (*Zhi Gan Cao*), 6g

2. Liver wind stirring internally

Symptoms: A red, numb, hypertonic tongue, inhibited speech, headache, dizziness, tinnitus, painful, distended eyes, possible clouded collapse, numb limbs, and unsteady steps in severe cases, and a wiry, fine pulse

Therapeutic principles: Level the liver and extinguish wind

Acupuncture & moxibustion:

Tong Li (Ht 5)
Lian Quan (CV 23)
Together, these points free the network vessels of the tongue.

Tai Chong (Liv 3)
Feng Chi (GB 20)
Together, these points level the liver and extinguish wind.

Ran Gu (Ki 2)
Nourishes yin and subdues yang

Additions and subtractions: For sudden collapse, add *Ren Zhong* (GV 26) and *Shi Xuan* (M-UE-1). For difficulty swallowing, add *Zhao Hai* (Ki 6) and *Tian Tu* (CV 22).

Chinese medicinal formula: *Zhen Gan Xi Feng Tang* (Settle the Liver & Extinguish Wind Decoction)

Ingredients: Uncooked Haemititum (*Dai Zhe Shi*), 18g, salt stir-fried Radix Achyranthis Bidentatae (*Niu Xi*), 18g, uncooked Os Draconis (*Long Gu*), 15g, uncooked Concha Ostreae (*Mu Li*), 15g, uncooked Plastrum Testudinis (*Gui Ban*), 15g, Radix Scrophulariae Ningpoensis (*Xuan Shen*), 9g, Tuber Asparagi Cochinensis (*Tian Men Dong*), 9g, uncooked Radix Albus Paeoniae Lactiflorae (*Bai Shao*), 15g, Herba Artemisiae Capillaris (*Yin Chen Hao*), 6g, Fructus Meliae Toosendan (*Chuan Lian Zi*), 6g, Fructus Germinatus Hordei Vulgaris (*Mai Ya*), 6g, Radix Glycyrrhizae (*Gan Cao*), 6g

3. Wind phlegm

Symptoms: A numb, hypertonic tongue, numb limbs, dizziness, vertigo, white, slimy tongue fur, and a wiry, slippery pulse

Therapeutic principles: Flush the phlegm and extinguish the wind

Acupuncture & moxibustion:

Tong Li (Ht 5)	Together, these points unblock the network vessels
Lian Quan (CV 23)	of the tongue.
Feng Fu (GV 16)	Together, these points extinguish the wind and can
Feng Chi (GB 20)	also dispel wind when there is concomitant external wind.
Feng Long (St 40)	Flushes the phlegm

Additions & subtractions: For numb limbs, add *Jian Yu* (LI 15), *Qu Chi* (LI 11), *He Gu* (LI 4), *Wai Guan* (TB 5), *Huan Tiao* (GB 30), *Yang Ling Quan* (GB 34), *Zu San Li* (St 36), *Jie Xi* (St 41), and *Kun Lun* (Bl 60) depending upon the symptoms. For deviated mouth and eyes, please refer to "Deviated Mouth & Eyes" in Volume 1 (p. 135-142).

Chinese medicinal formula: Modified *Dao Tan Tang* (Abduct the Phlegm Decoction) plus *Ban Xia Bai Zhu Tian Ma Tang* (Pinellia & Atractylodes, Gastrodia Decoction)

Ingredients: Lime-processed Rhizoma Pinelliae Ternatae (*Ban Xia*), 9g, bile-processed Rhizoma Arisaematis (*Dan Nan Xing*), 9g, Fructus Immaturus Citri Aurantii (*Zhi Shi*), 6g, Sclerotium Poriae Cocos (*Fu Ling*), 9g, Pericarpium Citri Reticulatae (*Chen Pi*), 9g, Rhizoma Gastrodiae Elatae (*Tian Ma*), 9g, uncooked Rhizoma Atractylodis Macrocephalae (*Bai Zhu*), 6g, mix-fried Radix Glycyrrhizae (*Zhi Gan*

Cao), 3g, Ramulus Uncariae Cum Uncis (*Gou Teng*), 9g, uncooked Concha Haliotidis (*Shi Jue Ming*), 30g

4. Phlegm fire

Symptoms: A numb, hypertonic tongue, dizziness, vertigo, cough with expectoration of thick, yellow phlegm, a bitter taste in the mouth, vexation, constipation, dark-colored urine, a red tongue with yellow, slimy fur, and a slippery, rapid pulse

Therapeutic principles: Clear heat and transform phlegm

Acupuncture & moxibustion:

Tong Li (Ht 5)	Together, these points unblock the network vessels
Jin Jin Yu Ye	of the tongue, and clear heart fire. Prick *Jin Jin*
(M-HN-20)	& *Yu Ye* to bleed.
Tai Chong (Liv 3)	Together, these points clear heat and transform
Yong Quan (Ki 1)	phlegm.
Feng Long (St 40)	
Ran Gu (Ki 2)	Protects yin to avoid damage to yin

Additions & subtractions: For constipation, add *Shang Ju Xu* (St 37) and *Tian Shu* (St 25).

Chinese medicinal formula: Modified *Qing Qi Hua Tan Wan* (Clear the Qi & Transform Phlegm Pills)

Ingredients: Fructus Trichosanthis Kirlowii (*Gua Lou*), 12g, uncooked Pericarpium Citri Reticulatae (*Chen Pi*), 9g, uncooked Radix Scutellariae Baicalensis (*Huang Qin*), 9g, Semen Pruni Armeniacae (*Xing Ren*), 9g, uncooked Fructus Immaturus Citri Aurantii (*Zhi Shi*), 9g, Sclerotium Poriae Cocos (*Fu Ling*), 9g, bile-processed Rhizoma Arisaematis (*Dan*

Nan Xing), 12g, lime-processed Rhizoma Pinelliae Ternatae (*Ban Xia*), 12g, Ramulus Uncariae Cum Uncis (*Gou Teng*), 9g, Rhizoma Coptidis Chinensis (*Huang Lian*), 6g, Buthus Martensi (*Quan Xie*), 3g, Bombyx Batryticatus (*Jiang Can*), 9g

Remarks: When numbness of the tongue is the main complaint, the most commonly seen pattern is blood vacuity. In this case, the important Chinese medicinals are Radix Albus Paeoniae Lactiflorae (*Bai Shao*), Radix Angelicae Sinensis (*Dang Gui*), and Caulis Milletiae Seu Spatholobi (*Ji Xue Teng*). Because qi vacuity is a frequent cause of blood vacuity, uncooked Radix Astragali Membranacei (*Huang Qi*) is also typically used. Uncooked Astragalus has a mobile nature. Therefore, it can infiltrate the vessels and network vessels, promoting the circulation of qi and blood in the vessels and tissues.

24
Limp Tongue (*She Wei*)

Limp tongue refers to a tongue which is flaccid and unable to move freely.

Disease causes, disease mechanisms:

I. Dual vacuity of qi & blood

This dual vacuity is mainly due to enduring disease and loss of blood which severely damages the heart and spleen. Being vacuous, the qi and blood cannot nourish the tongue and hence there is limp tongue.

2. Depletion of liver-kidney yin

This often occurs in the late stage of febrile disease where lingering evils or heat forcing the blood to move frenetically greatly damages liver and kidney yin. Once damaged, the essence, blood, and fluids and humors cannot irrigate the tongue. Therefore, there is limp tongue.

3. Heat evils fuming & burning

In the early stage of febrile disease, evils are often suppressed and then transforms into extreme heat in the qi division. Consumed by this heat, yin fluids then cannot sufficiently nourish the tongue. Thus limp tongue occurs.

4. Lung heat fuming & burning

Lung heat may be due to contraction of dry heat evils or uncleared heat that lingers in late stage febrile diseases. Heat can damage and consume fluids. If lung heat damages lung fluids to such an extent that these fluids fail to nourish the tongue network vessels, limp tongue will occur.

5. Phlegm dampness blocking the network vessels

Phlegm dampness can be the result of abnormality in the function of the lungs, kidneys, and especially of the spleen. Since these are the three viscera which govern water metabolism in the body, they are the ones most closely associated with the formation of dampness. If dampness arises, it may accumulate and then become phlegm if it congeals over time. If phlegm dampness moves upward and blocks the channel and network vessels of the tongue, the flow of qi and blood and the qi mechanism will be affected, leading to less nourishment and inhibition of the qi mechanism. Hence there will be a limp tongue.

Treatment based on pattern discrimination:

I. Dual vacuity of the qi & blood

Symptoms: A limp tongue that cannot move efficiently, a white, lusterless facial complexion, pale white lips and nails, low voice while speaking, heart palpitations and racing heart, fatigued limbs, insomnia, impaired memory, reduced food intake, a pale, tender tongue with thin, white fur, and a fine, forceless pulse

Therapeutic principles: Boost the heart and spleen, supplement the qi and blood

Acupuncture & moxibustion:

Lian Quan (CV 23)   Boosts the tongue

Shen Men (Ht 7) *San Yin Jiao* (Sp 6)	Together, these points supplement the heart and spleen.
He Gu (LI 4) *Zu San Li* (St 36)	Together, these points boost the qi.

Chinese medicinal formula: Modified *Gui Pi Tang* (Return the Spleen Decoction)

Ingredients: Honey stir-fried Radix Astragali Membranacei (*Huang Qi*), 15g, bran stir-fried Rhizoma Atractylodis Macrocephalae (*Bai Zhu*), 9g, stir-fried Radix Angelicae Sinensis (*Dang Gui*), 12g, Sclerotium Poriae Cocos (*Fu Ling*), 9g, Radix Auklandiae Lappae (*Mu Xiang*), 3g, mix-fried Radix Glycyrrhizae (*Zhi Gan Cao*), 3g, Radix Codonopsitis Pilosulae (*Dang Shen*), 9g, Arillus Euphoriae Longanae (*Long Yan Rou*), 6g, stir-fried Semen Zizyphi Spinosae (*Suan Zao Ren*), 9g, Radix Albus Paeoniae Lactiflorae (*Bai Shao*), 9g

2. Depletion of liver-kidney yin

Symptoms: A dull, limp tongue, cloudedness and somnolence, fatigued spirit, red cheekbones, dry mouth and teeth, deafness, low fever, trembling fingers, racing heart, a purple tongue with no fur, and a vacuous, soft, or bound or regularly interrupted pulse

Therapeutic principles: Enrich and nourish the liver and kidneys

Acupuncture & moxibustion:

Lian Quan (CV 23)	Boosts the tongue
San Yin Jiao (Sp 6) *Qu Quan* (Liv 8) *Tai Xi* (Ki 3)	Together, these points enrich and nourish the liver and kidneys when needled with supplementing method.

Tai Chong (Liv 3)	Levels the liver when needled with slightly draining method.

Additions & subtractions: For persistent low fever and night sweats, add *Fu Liu* (Ki 7).

Chinese medicinal formula: *Jia Wei Fu Mai Tang* (Added Restore the Pulse Decoction)

Ingredients: Uncooked Radix Rehmanniae (*Sheng Di*), 15g, uncooked Radix Albus Paeoniae Lactiflorae (*Bai Shao*), 15g, Tuber Ophiopogonis Japonici (*Mai Men Dong*), 12g, Gelatinum Corii Asini (*E Jiao*), 6g, Semen Cannabis Sativae (*Huo Ma Ren*), 6g, mix-fried Radix Glycyrrhizae (*Zhi Gan Cao*), 3g, steamed Fructus Corni Officinalis (*Shan Zhu Yu*), 12g, vinegar dip-calcined Plastrum Testudinis (*Gui Ban*), 15g

3. Heat evils fuming & burning

Symptoms: A red, limp, dry tongue, fever, vexation, thirst, short voidings of dark-colored urine, dry stool, and a fine, rapid pulse

Therapeutic principles: Clear heat, engender fluids, and free the bowels

Acupuncture & moxibustion:

Tong Li (Ht 5)	Together, these points clear local heat and heat in
Lian Quan (CV 23)	the heart to disinhibit the portal.
Jian Shi (Per 5)	

Tian Shu (St 25)	Together, these points engender fluids to "increase
San Yin Jiao (Sp 6)	the water and sail the boat" so as to clear heat.
Fu Liu (Ki 7)	

Additions & subtractions: For constipation, add *Tian Shu* (St 25). For drooling, add *Di Cang* (St 4) and *Cheng Jiang* (CV 24).

Chinese medicinal formula: *Xie Xin Tang* (Drain the Heart Decoction)

Ingredients: Uncooked Radix Scutellariae Baicalensis (*Huang Qin*), 9g, wine stir-fried Rhizoma Coptidis Chinensis (*Huang Lian*), 6g, uncooked Radix Et Rhizoma Rhei (*Da Huang*), 6-9g, Rhizoma Anemarrhenae Asphodeloidis (*Zhi Mu*), 9g, Folium Bambusae (*Zhu Ye*), 9g

4. Lung heat fuming & burning

Symptoms: A dry, limp tongue, dry cough with no expectoration or scanty, sticky phlegm, qi counterflow panting, dry throat and nose, vexation, thirst, short voidings of dark-colored urine, dry stool or uneasy defecation, a red tongue with thin, yellow fur and reduced fluids, and a fine, rapid pulse

Therapeutic principles: Clear the lungs, nourish yin, and moisten dryness

Acupuncture & moxibustion:

Lian Quan (CV 23)   Clears local heat and engenders fluids

Chi Ze (Lu 5)   Together, these points clear heat to protect fluids.
Nei Ting (St 44)

Fu Liu (Ki 7)   Nourishes yin and moistens dryness

Additions & subtractions: For severe panting, add *Shan Zhong* (CV 17) and *Tian Tu* (CV 22). For severe vexation, add *Shen Men* (Ht 7).

Chinese medicinal formula: *Qing Zao Jiu Fei Tang* (Clear Dryness & Rescue the Lungs Decoction)

Ingredients: Honey mix-fried Folium Mori Albi (*Sang Ye*), 9g, uncooked Gypsum Fibrosum (*Shi Gao*), 12g, uncooked Radix Codonopsitis Pilosulae (*Dang Shen*), 6g, Radix Glycyrrhizae (*Gan Cao*), 3g, Semen Lini (*Hu Ma Ren*), 6g, Gelatinum Corii Asini (*E Jiao*), 6g, Tuber

Ophiopogonis Japonici (*Mai Men Dong*), 6g, Semen Pruni Armeniacae (*Xing Ren*), 6g, Folium Eriobotryae Japonicae (*Pi Pa Ye*), 6g

5. Phlegm dampness blocking the network vessels

Symptoms: A limp tongue with inability to move, inhibited speech, a white facial complexion, blue lips, glomus and oppression in the chest and stomach, vomiting or nausea, encumbered limbs, heart palpitations, dizziness, vertigo, a pale red tongue with thick, glossy, slimy fur, and a deep, slippery pulse

Therapeutic principles: Fortify the spleen and dry dampness, flush the phlegm and open the portal

Acupuncture & moxibustion:

Tong Li (Ht 5)	Together, these points unblock the network vessels
Lian Quan (CV 23)	of the tongue to open the portal.

He Gu (LI 4)	Together, these points fortify the spleen and dry
Zu San Li (St 36)	dampness as well as move the qi to transform phlegm.

Feng Long (St 40)	Flushes phlegm

Chinese medicinal formula: Modified *Di Tan Tang* (Flush Phlegm Decoction)

Ingredients: Lime-processed Rhizoma Pinelliae Ternatae (*Ban Xia*), 9g, bile-processed Rhizoma Arisaematis (*Dan Nan Xing*), 9g, Pericarpium Citri Reticulatae (*Chen Pi*), 6g, Fructus Immaturus Citri Aurantii (*Zhi Shi*), 6g, Sclerotium Poriae Cocos (*Fu Ling*), 9g, Radix Codonopsitis Pilosulae (*Dang Shen*), 6g, Caulis Bambusae In Taeniis (*Zhu Ru*), 6g, Rhizoma Acori Graminei (*Shi Chang Pu*), 9g, uncooked Rhizoma

Zingiberis (*Sheng Jiang*), 3g, Radix Glycyrrhizae (*Gan Cao*), 3g, uncooked Rhizoma Typhonii Gigantei (*Bai Fu Zi*), 6g

25
Painful Tongue (*She Tong*)

Painful tongue refers to the subjective sensation of burning, stabbing, etc. in the tongue. This pain may be felt in the whole tongue body or on only the tip, edge, or the center of the tongue. Pain which is secondary to a tongue sore is not dealt with herein.

Disease causes, disease mechanisms:

1. Replete heat of the viscera & bowels

This heat is often engendered internally from dietary irregularities and excesses of the five affects. Most of the viscera and bowels have, in one way or another, a connection with the tongue. If replete heat flares upward along the channels to the tongue, pain in the tongue may occur.

2. Yin vacuity, fire effulgence

Yin vacuity may arise from enduring disease, lifestyle irregularities, and during the late stage of febrile diseases which consume yin. If there is yin vacuity, yang will be unchecked, resulting in fire effulgence. If this yin vacuity fire flares upward along the channels, there may be pain in the tongue.

Treatment based on pattern discrimination:

I. Heart fire flaming upward

Symptoms: Pricking pain at the tip of the tongue accompanied by vexation, dark-colored urine, possible painful urination, a red tongue tip, and a rapid pulse

Therapeutic principles: Clear the heart and drain fire

Acupuncture & moxibustion:

Lian Quan (CV 23)	Clears heat locally and stops pain by freeing the flow of qi
Da Ling (Per 7) *Shen Men* (Ht 7)	Together, these points clear the heart and drain fire.
Zhong Ji (CV 3)	Disinhibits urination to drain the fire from the urine

Additions & subtractions: For a bitter taste in the mouth, add *Yang Ling Quan* (GB 34) and *Lao Gong* (Per 8).

Chinese medicinal formula: Modified *Dao Chi San* (Abduct the Red Decoction)

Ingredients: Uncooked Radix Rehmanniae (*Sheng Di*), 12g, Caulis Akebiae (*Mu Tong*), 6g, Cacumen Glycyrrhizae (*Gan Cao Shao*), 6g, Herba Lophatheri Gracilis (*Dan Zhu Ye*), 3g, Rhizoma Coptidis Chinensis (*Huang Lian*), 6g

2. Liver-gallbladder fire attacking upward

Symptoms: Pain and redness on the sides of the tongue accompanied by a bitter taste in the mouth, vexation and irascibility, possible red eyes, and a wiry, rapid pulse

Therapeutic principles: Clear and drain the liver and gallbladder

Acupuncture & moxibustion:

Lian Quan (CV 23)
Tong Li (Ht 5)

Together, these points clear heat in the local area and stop pain.

Xing Jian (Liv 2)
Xia Xi (GB 43)
Qiu Xu (GB 40)

Together, these points clear and drain the liver and gallbladder when needled with draining method.

Additions & subtractions: For distended eyes, prick *Tong Zi Liao* (GB 1) to bleed. For dizziness and vertigo, add *Feng Chi* (GB 20).

Chinese medicinal formula: Modified *Long Dan Xie Gan Tang* (Gentiana Drain the Liver Decoction)

Ingredients: Radix Gentianae Scabrae (*Long Dan Cao*), 9g, uncooked Radix Scutellariae Baicalensis (*Huang Qin*), 9g, uncooked Fructus Gardeniae Jasminoidis (*Zhi Zi*), 6g, Caulis Akebiae (*Mu Tong*), 6g, Semen Plantaginis (*Che Qian Zi*), 6g, uncooked Radix Angelicae Sinensis (*Dang Gui*), 6g, uncooked Radix Rehmanniae (*Sheng Di*), 6g, uncooked Radix Bupleuri (*Chai Hu*), 3g

Additions & subtractions: If there is constipation, add uncooked Radix Et Rhizoma Rhei (*Da Huang*), 6g, or Herba Aloes (*Lu Hui*), 1g (powder and take with the strained decoction).

3. Stomach fire flaming upward

Symptoms: Pain in the center of the tongue accompanied by painful, swollen gums, thirst with a liking for chilled drinks, poor appetite, constipation, dry, yellow tongue fur, and a rapid or slippery, rapid pulse

Therapeutic principles: Clear the stomach and drain fire

Acupuncture & moxibustion:

Jin Jin Yu Ye (M-HN-20)	When pricked to bleed, clears heat in the local area.
Shang Lian Quan (M-HN-21)	Helps the above point clear heat and stops pain
Jie Xi (St 41) *Nei Ting* (St 44)	Together, these points clear the stomach and drain fire when needled with draining method.
Fu Liu (Ki 7)	Protects yin when needled with supplementing method

Additions & subtractions: For bad breath, add *Lao Gong* (Per 8).

Chinese medicinal formula: Modified *Qing Wei San* (Clear Stomach Powder)

Ingredients: Uncooked Gypsum Fibrosum (*Shi Gao*), 15g, wine stir-fried Rhizoma Coptidis Chinensis (*Huang Lian*), 6g, uncooked Radix Rehmanniae (*Sheng Di*), 12g, uncooked Radix Angelicae Sinensis (*Dang Gui*), 9g, Cortex Radicis Moutan (*Dan Pi*), 6g, uncooked Rhizoma Cimicifugae (*Sheng Ma*), 6g, Radix Glycyrrhizae (*Gan Cao*), 3g

Additions & subtractions: If there is constipation, add uncooked Radix Et Rhizoma Rhei (*Da Huang*), 9g, and Mirabilitum (*Mang Xiao*), 6g.

4. Lung fire fuming & burning

Symptoms: Painful tongue with an acrid taste in the mouth accompanied by dry throat and nose, dry cough with scanty or no phlegm, thirst, short voidings of dark-colored urine, a red tongue with yellow fur lacking fluids, and a rapid or fine, rapid pulse

Therapeutic principles: Clear the lungs and drain fire

Acupuncture & moxibustion:

Lian Quan (CV 23) *Yi Feng* (TB 17)	Together, these points clear heat in the local area. In addition, *Yi Feng* can free the triple burner channel to clear the heat in the upper burner.
Shao Shang (Lu 11) *Yu Ji* (Lu 10) *Chi Ze* (Lu 5)	Together, these points clear the lungs and drain fire. In addition, *Chi Ze* also protects yin.

Additions & subtractions: For cough, add *Fei Shu* (Bl 13) and *Tian Tu* (CV 22).

Chinese medicinal formula: Modified *Xie Bai San* (Drain the White Powder)

Ingredients: Cortex Radicis Mori Albi (*Sang Bai Pi*), 9g, Cortex Radicis Lycii Chinensis (*Di Gu Pi*), 6g, Radix Glycyrrhizae (*Gan Cao*), 9g, uncooked Radix Scutellariae Baicalensis (*Huang Qin*), 9g, uncooked Radix Platycodi Grandiflori (*Jie Geng*), 9g, Tuber Ophiopogonis Japonici (*Mai Men Dong*), 6g, Fructus Trichosanthis Kirlowii (*Gua Lou*), 9g, Bulbus Fritillariae Cirrhosae (*Chuan Bei Mu*), 9g, Rhizoma Anemarrhenae Asphodeloidis (*Zhi Mu*), 6g

5. Phlegm fire attacking upward

Symptoms: Pain and numbness in the tongue accompanied by glomus and fullness in the chest and stomach, possible inhibited speech, encumbered limbs, a red tongue with yellow, thick, slimy fur, and a rapid, slippery pulse

Therapeutic principles: Clear fire and flush the phlegm

Acupuncture & moxibustion:

Jin Jin Yu Ye (M-HN-20) *Lian Quan* (CV 23)	Together, these points clear fire and sweep away the phlegm from the local area to stop pain and disinhibit the portal.
Xian Gu (St 43) *Feng Long* (St 40) *Yin Ling Quan* (Sp 9)	Together, these points clear heat and flush phlegm.

Chinese medicinal formula: *Meng Shi Gun Tan Wan* (Mica Roll Phlegm Pills)

Ingredients: Uncooked Radix Et Rhizoma Rhei (*Da Huang*), 240g, uncooked Radix Scutellariae Baicalensis (*Huang Qin*), 240g, Lapis Micae Seu Chloriti (*Meng Shi*), 30g, Lignum Aquilariae Agallochae (*Chen Xiang*), 15g

Method of use: Powder the above medicinals and make into pills with water. Take 5-9g each time, 2 times per day with warm water.

6. Heat toxins of the viscera & bowels

Symptoms: Pain in the whole tongue accompanied by thirst, vexation, a bitter taste in the mouth, insomnia, constipation, short voidings of dark-colored urine, possible painful urination, a red tongue with yellow fur, and a rapid or fine, rapid pulse

Therapeutic principles: Clear heat and resolve toxins

Acupuncture & moxibustion:

Jin Jin Yu Ye (M-HN-20)	Clears heat and resolves toxins when pricked to bleed
Shi Xuan (M-UE-1)	Clears heat and resolves toxins of the viscera and bowels

Use the above group of points alternately with the following group: *Lian Quan* (CV 23), *Yong Quan* (Ki 1), *Xia Xi* (GB 43), *Xing Jian* (Liv 2) and *Nei Ting* (St 44).

Chinese medicinal formula: Modified *Huang Lian Jie Du Tang* (Coptis Resolve Toxins Decoction)

Ingredients: Wine stir-fried Rhizoma Coptidis Chinensis (*Huang Lian*), 6g, uncooked Radix Scutellariae Baicalensis (*Huang Qin*), 6g, uncooked Cortex Phellodendri (*Huang Bai*), 6g, uncooked Fructus Gardeniae Jasminoidis (*Zhi Zi*), 9g, uncooked Radix Et Rhizoma Rhei (*Da Huang*), 6g

7. Heart yin vacuity with effulgent fire

Symptoms: A red, burning tongue with reduced or no fur, insomnia, sleep with profuse dreaming, vexation, vexatious heat in the five hearts, heart palpitations and racing heart, and a fine, rapid pulse

Therapeutic principles: Nourish yin, supplement the heart, and quiet the spirit

Acupuncture & moxibustion:

Lian Quan (CV 23)	Clears heat in the local area and stops pain

Shen Men (Ht 7)	Together, these points clear the heart. In addition,
Da Ling (Per 7)	*Shen Men* can also nourish heart yin.

Fu Liu (Ki 7)	Together, these points nourish yin so that water
San Yin Jiao (Sp 6)	helps the fire above.

Chinese medicinal formula: Modified *Tian Wang Bu Xin Dan* (Heavenly Emperor Supplement the Heart Elixir)

Ingredients: Uncooked Radix Rehmanniae (*Sheng Di*), 9g, Radix Panacis Ginseng (*Ren Shen*), 6g, Tuber Asparagi Cochinensis (*Tian Men Dong*), 6g, Tuber Ophiopogonis Japonici (*Mai Men Dong*), 9g, Radix Scrophulariae Ningpoensis (*Xuan Shen*), 3g, Radix Salviae Miltiorrhizae (*Dan Shen*), 6g, Sclerotium Poriae Cocos (*Fu Ling*), 6g, Radix Polygalae Tenuifoliae (*Yuan Zhi*), 9g, Radix Angelicae Sinensis (*Dang Gui*), 6g, Fructus Schisandrae Chinensis (*Wu Wei Zi*), 9g, Semen Biotae Orientalis (*Bai Zi Ren*), 9g, stir-fried Semen Zizyphi Spinosae (*Suan Zao Ren*), 9g, Radix Platycodi Grandiflori (*Jie Geng*), 3g

8. Kidney yin vacuity with effulgent fire

Symptoms: A painful, dry tongue with reduced or no fur, dry mouth and throat, insomnia, tinnitus, night sweats, pain and weakness of the low back and knees, and a fine, rapid pulse

Therapeutic principles: Enrich the kidneys and nourish yin

Acupuncture & moxibustion:

Lian Quan (CV 23)	Engenders fluids and stops pain in the tongue

Shen Men (Ht 7)	Clears the heart to interact with the kidneys

Tai Xi (Ki 3)	Together, these points enrich the kidneys and
Fu Liu (Ki 7)	nourish yin.
San Yin Jiao (Sp 6)	

Additions & subtractions: For seminal emission, add *Yin Gu* (Ki 10). For sore throat, add *Zhao Hai* (Ki 6).

Chinese medicinal formula: *Liu Wei Di Huang Wan* (Six Flavors Rehmannia Pills)

Ingredients: Prepared Radix Rehmanniae (*Shu Di*), 24g, steamed Fructus Corni Officinalis (*Shan Zhu Yu*), 12g, stir-fried Radix Dioscoreae Oppositae (*Shan Yao*), 12g, Sclerotium Poriae Cocos (*Fu Ling*), 6g, Cortex Radicis Moutan (*Dan Pi*), 6g, Rhizoma Alismatis (*Ze Xie*), 6g

26
Curled Tongue (*She Juan*)

Curled tongue refers to a tongue that is curled and shortened with inhibited movement and delirious speech.

Disease causes, disease mechanisms:

I. Depletion of liver channel qi

This is often encountered in severe disease where evils enter the liver channel and transform into exuberant heat, burning and consuming yin fluids. Yin and yang are mutually dependent. If liver yin becomes depleted, yang depletion will follow. "The liver governs the sinews." If the liver channel qi is depleted, the sinews will lose their control, and therefore, there is curled tongue.

2. Heat falling inward to the pericardium

In warm disease, heat may be transmitted to the pericardium which takes the evils in the place of the heart. The heart has its effloresence in the tongue. If the heart is attacked by heat and the spirit is harassed, there may be curled tongue and delirious speech.

Treatment based on pattern discrimination:

I. Depletion of liver channel qi

Symptoms: Curled tongue, shrinking of the scrotum, cramping, clouded spirit, vexation, fullness in the chest, blue lips, a red crimson tongue with reduced fluids, and a wiry, rapid pulse

Therapeutic principles: Clear heat and extinguish wind

Acupuncture & moxibustion:

Lian Quan (CV 23)	Together, these points clear heat and relax the
Tian Tu (CV 22)	tongue.

Qu Gu (CV 2)	Together, these points enrich yin and clear heat,
Shen Shu (Bl 23)	extinguish wind and soothe the sinews.
Fu Liu (Ki 7)	
Ran Gu (KI 3)	
Xue Hai (Sp 10)	

Chinese medicinal formula: Modified *Ling Yang Jiao Gou Teng Tang* (Antelope Horn & Gastrodia Decoction)

Ingredients: Cornu Caprae (*Shan Yang Jiao*), 15g, Ramulus Uncariae Cum Uncis (*Gou Teng*), 12g, Caulis Bambusae In Taeniis (*Zhu Ru*), 6g, uncooked Radix Rehmanniae (*Sheng Di*), 15g, Folium Mori Albi (*Sang Ye*), 9g, Bulbus Fritillariae Thunbergii (*Zhe Bei Mu*), 6g, Flos Chrysanthemi Morifolii (*Ju Hua*), 15g, Sclerotium Pararadicis Poriae Cocos (*Fu Shen*), 9g, Radix Albus Paeoniae Lactiflorae (*Bai Shao*), 12g, Radix Glycyrrhizae (*Gan Cao*), 3g, uncooked Concha Haliotidis (*Shi Jue Ming*), 15g, uncooked Carapax Amydae Sinensis (*Bie Jia*), 12g, Carapax Eretmochelios (*Dai Mao*), 12g

2. Heat falling inward to the pericardium

Symptoms: Curled tongue, high fever, red cheekbones, counterflow chilling of the limbs, constipation, a red crimson tongue, and a surging, rapid or wiry, slippery, rapid pulse

Therapeutic principles: Clear heat and resolve toxins, cool the blood and unblock the portals

Acupuncture & moxibustion:

Jin Jin Yu Ye (M-HN-20) *Shi Xuan* (M-UE-1)	Together, when pricked to bleed, these points clear the heart and resolve the toxins, cool the blood and open the portals.

Additions & subtractions: For vexation and agitation, add *Shen Men* (Ht 7). For high fever, add *Da Zhui* (GV 14). For coma, add *Ren Zhong* (GV 26) or *Su Liao* (GV 25).

Chinese medicinal formula: Modified *An Gong Niu Huang Wan* (Quiet the Palace Bezoar Pills)

Ingredients: Calculus Bovis (*Niu Huang*), 0.5g (not decocted), Tuber Curcumae (*Yu Jin*), 9g, Cornu Bubali (*Shui Niu Jiao*), 30g, Rhizoma Coptidis Chinensis (*Huang Lian*), 9g, Cinnabar (*Zhu Sha*), 0.5g (not decocted), Borneol (*Bing Pian*), 0.5g (not decocted), Secretio Moschi Moschiferi (*She Xiang*), 0.05g (not decocted), Margarita (*Zhen Zhu*), 0.5g (powdered), Fructus Gardeniae Jasminoidis (*Zhi Zi*), 9g, Realgar (*Xiong Huang*), 0.5g (not decocted), Radix Scutellariae Baicalensis (*Huang Qin*), 9g

Method of use: Decoct the Curcuma, water buffalo horn, Coptis, Scutellaria, and Gardenia first. Then take the other ingredients washed down with the warm decoction. The above dosage is for one day.

27
Dry Tongue (*She Gan*)

Dry tongue refers to a tongue which lacks moisture and feels rough. Breathing through the mouth due to nasal congestion can also cause dry tongue, but this is not discussed herein.

Disease causes, disease mechanisms:

1. Exuberant heat damaging fluids

In warm disease, warm evils often give rise to heat exuberance, resulting in damage to the fluids. When the fluids are damaged so severely that they cannot moisten the tongue sufficiently, there will be a dry tongue.

2. Yin vacuity & liquid exhaustion

Yin liquid vacuity can arise from late stage febrile disease where heat evils linger and consume yin liquid. It may also be due to enduring disease where yin is consumed little by little, day by day. In that case, yin vacuity fire may occur which damages yin liquid even further. If yin liquid is damaged to such an extent that it cannot provide sufficient moisture to the tongue, a dry tongue will occur.

3. Vacuous yang failing to upbear fluids

Yang vacuity may be due to enduring disease, aging, unrestrained sexual activity, or sudden and massive loss of yin fluids with which yang is lost simultaneously (*i.e.*, blood and yin desertion leading to qi and yang desertion). Yang is supposed to transform and distribute fluids. If yang is vacuous, yang cannot transform and distribute the fluids properly. If yang fails to upbear the fluids to moisten the tongue, there will be a dry tongue.

Treatment based on pattern discrimination:

1. Exuberant heat damaging fluids

Symptoms: A dry tongue with dry, yellow fur and possible prickles, high fever, a red face, vexation and agitation, thirst with a desire for chilled drinks, profuse sweating, short voidings of dark-colored urine, and a surging, rapid pulse

Therapeutic principles: Clear heat and engender fluids

Acupuncture & moxibustion:

Jin Jin Yu Ye (M-HN-20) Engenders fluids when pricked to bleed

Fei Shu (Bl 13) Together, these points clear heat and engender
Chi Ze (Lu 5) fluids.
Shen Men (Ht 7)

Fu Liu (Ki 7) Nourishes yin and stops sweating

Chinese medicinal formula: *Bai Hu Jia Ren Shen Tang* (White Tiger & Ginseng Decoction)

Ingredients: Uncooked Gypsum Fibrosum (*Shi Gao*), 30g, uncooked Rhizoma Anemarrhenae Asphodeloidis (*Zhi Mu*), 9g, Radix Glycyrrhizae (*Gan Cao*), 6g, Semen Oryzae Sativae (*Geng Mi*), 9g, white Radix Panacis Ginseng (*Bai Ren Shen*), 9g

2. Yin vacuity & liquid exhaustion

Symptoms: A red, dry tongue with reduced or no fur, dry mouth and throat, fever worse at night, tidal flushing of the face, heat in the palms of the hands and soles of the feet, short voidings of dark-colored urine, and a fine, rapid pulse

Therapeutic principles: Enrich yin and increase liquids

Acupuncture & moxibustion:

Lian Quan (CV 23)	Engenders fluids
Shao Ze (SI 1) *Qu Ze* (Per 3)	Together, these points increase liquids and also clear heat.
Tai Xi (Ki 3) *Fu Liu* (Ki 7) *Gan Shu* (Bl 18)	Together, these points enrich yin and downbear fire.

Chinese medicinal formula: Modified *Zeng Ye Tang* (Increase Fluids Decoction)

Ingredients: Radix Scrophulariae Ningpoensis (*Xuan Shen*), 9g, Tuber Ophiopogonis Japonici (*Mai Men Dong*), 9g, uncooked Radix Rehmanniae (*Sheng Di*), 9g, Rhizoma Phragmitis Communis (*Lu Gen*), 9g, Radix Trichosanthis Kirlowii (*Tian Hua Fen*), 9g, Herba Dendrobii (*Shi Hu*), 9g, Radix Glycyrrhizae (*Gan Cao*), 6g

3. Vacuous yang failing to upbear fluids[8]

Symptoms: A pale, dry tongue with white fur, thirst with no desire to drink or with a desire for hot drinks, a bright pale or dull facial

---

[8] Usually, for thirst or a dry tongue, we think replete or vacuity heat. However, this pattern is not rare but, in fact, is commonly met. In this case, thirst or a dry tongue are due to spleen qi or yang vacuity typically complicated by damp accumulation. The main cause of this is dietary irregularities, such as chilled and uncooked foods, ice cream, cold drinks, etc. In case of spleen qi and yang vacuity, Ramulus Cinnamomi Cassiae (*Gui Zhi*) and Rhizoma Atractylodis Macrocephalae (*Bai Zhu*) are the key Chinese medicinals. In case of damp accumulation, Sclerotium Poriae Cocos (*Fu Ling*) and Rhizoma Pinelliae Ternatae (*Ban Xia*) are the key Chinese medicinals.

complexion, fatigue and lack of strength, limbs lacking warmth, clear urine, loose stools, puffy edema, and a deep, slow pulse

Therapeutic principles: Warm yang and disinhibit water

Acupuncture & moxibustion:

Lian Quan (CV 23)	Quickens the network vessels in the local area

Bai Hui (GV 20)	Together, when moxaed, these points warm yang.
Guan Yuan (CV 4)	
Qi Hai (CV 6)	

Zu San Li (St 36)	Together, these points fortify the spleen, boost the
San Yin Jiao (Sp 6)	qi, and disinhibit water.

Chinese medicinal formula: Modified *Zhen Wu Tang* (True Warrior Decoction)

Ingredients: Bland Radix Lateralis Praeparatus Aconiti Carmichaeli (*Fu Zi*), 6g, uncooked Rhizoma Atractylodis Macrocephalae (*Bai Zhu*), 9g, Radix Albus Paeoniae Lactiflorae (*Bai Shao*), 6g, uncooked Rhizoma Zingiberis (*Sheng Jiang*), 9g, Sclerotium Poriae Cocos (*Fu Ling*), 9g, Semen Plantaginis (*Che Qian Zi*), 6g, stir-fried Ramulus Cinnamomi Cassiae (*Gui Zhi*), 9g, honey stir-fried Radix Astragali Membranacei (*Huang Qi*), 15g

28
Fissured Tongue (*She Lie*)

A fissured tongue refers to clefts of different depths and shapes on the surface of the tongue.

Disease causes, disease mechanisms:

A fissured tongue is due, in one word, to yin blood vacuity that fails to nourish and moisten the tongue.

I. Replete heat in the *yang ming*

In febrile disease, when heat enters the *yang ming* and binds there, it will burn and damage fluids and liquids. If they become damaged, the fluids and liquid cannot nourish and moisten the tongue. Therefore, there is a fissured tongue.

2. Yin vacuity & liquid exhaustion

Yin vacuity and liquid exhaustion are mainly due to enduring disease that consumes yin or to late stage warm disease where evils linger, burn, and damage yin liquid. When yin liquid is severely damaged and cannot nourish and moisten the tongue, there is a fissured tongue.

Treatment based on pattern discrimination:

Though many symptoms can help in the pattern discrimination of this condition, the most significant one is whether or not there is tongue fur.

I. Replete heat in the *yang ming*

Symptoms: A fissured tongue with yellow, dry fur, tidal fever, thirst with a desire for drinking a lot, delirium, abdominal fullness and pain that refuses pressure, sweating from the hands and feet, aversion to heat, vexation and agitation, constipation, and a surging, rapid or deep, replete pulse

Acupuncture & moxibustion:

Jin Jin Yu Ye (M-HN-20)	Clears heat and engenders fluids when pricked to bleed
Tian Shu (St 25) *Shui Dao* (St 28) *Shang Ju Xu* (St 37)	Together, these points free the bowels to protect yin.
Shang Yang (LI 1) *Li Dui* (St 45)	Together, these points drain fire when pricked to bleed.

Additions & subtractions: If there is still constipation, add *Zhi Gou* (TB 6) with draining method and *Zhao Hai* (Ki 6) with supplementing method.

Chinese medicinal formula: *Da Cheng Qi Tang* (Major Order the Qi Decoction)

Ingredients: Uncooked Radix Et Rhizoma Rhei (*Da Huang*), 9g, Mirabilitum (*Mang Xiao*), 6g, uncooked Fructus Immaturus Citri Aurantii (*Zhi Shi*), 6g, ginger mix-fried Cortex Magnoliae Officinalis (*Hou Po*), 9g

2. Yin vacuity & liquid exhaustion

Symptoms: Fissures on the surface of the tongue with no tongue fur, thirst, vexatious heat in the five hearts, emaciation, a red, crimson tongue with reduced fluids, and a fine, rapid pulse

Therapeutic principles: Enrich yin and clear heat

Acupuncture and moxibustion:

Lian Quan (CV 23)	Engenders fluids
Ye Men (TB 2) *Zhao Hai* (Ki 6)	Together, these points engender fluids and clear heat.
San Yin Jiao (Sp 6) *Tai Xi* (Ki 3)	Together, these points enrich yin and downbear fire.

Additions & subtractions: For insomnia, add *Shen Men* (Ht 7).

Chinese medicinal formula: Modified *Zeng Ye Tang* (Increase Fluids Decoction)

Ingredients: Radix Scrophulariae Ningpoensis (*Xuan Shen*), 9g, Tuber Ophiopogonis Japonici (*Mai Men Dong*), 9g, uncooked Radix Rehmanniae (*Sheng Di*), 9g, Rhizoma Phragmitis Communis (*Lu Gen*), 9g, Radix Trichosanthis Kirlowii (*Tian Hua Fen*), 9g, Herba Dendrobii (*Shi Hu*), 9g, Radix Glycyrrhizae (*Gan Cao*), 6g

Remarks: The above discussion of fissured tongue assumes that the tongue is also red in color. However, various types of cracks on the tongue when the tongue is not red in color do not necessarily mean there is a fluid insufficiency. For instance, many small, shallow cracks on the middle surface of the tongue, a centerline crack with branching horizontal cracks, and horizontal cracks on the sides of the tongue all indicate prolonged spleen vacuity. In fact, as long as the tongue is not red and there are no marked symptoms of yin vacuity heat and dryness, shallow cracks on the surface of the tongue are an important indicator of spleen vacuity.

In such cases, the practitioner is advised to look for signs of stomach heat and/or dryness, since frequently in clinical practice, the spleen will become vacuous and damp while the stomach will become hot and dry. Symptoms of stomach heat and dryness include rapid hungering and large food intake, thirst, pimples along the course of the *yang ming* on the face, and floating pulse in the right *guan* position. However, if there is a centerline crack with branching horizontal cracks or horizontal cracks on the sides of the tongue, this usually indicates more serious spleen and stomach vacuity with possible cold and less likely stomach heat.

A broad centerline crack with yellow fur inside suggests phlegm heat accompanied by underlying spleen vacuity. And two diagonal cracks in the area of the lungs on the front third of the tongue can indicate that the lungs have been damaged by chronic disease in the past, for instance due to pediatric asthma and chronic bronchitis.

29
Spontaneous Bleeding of the Tongue (*She Nu*)

Spontaneous bleeding of the tongue refers to needle-eye-sized openings on the tongue from which the blood oozes out.

Disease causes, disease mechanisms:

1. Exuberant heart fire

This heat can be from excesses of the five affects that transform heat, contraction of external evils entering the interior and then transforming into heat, addiction to alcohol or rich, spicy food that engenders heat, or from enduring administration or overdosage of warm, supplementing agents. If exuberant heat flames upward along the channel, burns and damages the network vessels of the tongue, and forces the blood to move frenetically, there will be spontaneous bleeding from the tongue.

2. Yin vacuity fire flaring upward

Yin vacuity fire may be due to a yin vacuity constitution, febrile disease which burns and damages true yin, unrestrained sexual activity, or to loss of blood, essence, and/or liquid. If yin vacuity fire flares upward along the channels to the tongue, it may burn and damage the network vessels in the tongue, leading to spontaneous bleeding from the tongue.

3. Spleen failing to contain the blood

The spleen is responsible for containing the blood. Therefore, if there is spleen qi vacuity due to constitutional insufficiency, taxation, over-thinking, dietary irregularities, or wrongful administration of cold and cool agents which damage spleen yang, the spleen may fail to contain the blood. This then may lead to spontaneous bleeding from the tongue since the tongue is rich in network vessels.

Treatment based on pattern discrimination:

I. Exuberant heart fire

Symptoms: Persistent bleeding from the tongue which is profuse in amount, a painful, swollen tongue with a red crimson tongue tip and possible prickles, vexatious heat in the heart, a red face, thirst with desire to drink, astringent voidings of dark-colored urine, insomnia, sleep with profuse dreaming, possible delirium, and a rapid, forceful pulse

Therapeutic principles: Clear the heart and drain fire

Acupuncture & moxibustion:

Zhong Chong (Per 9) *Wai Guan* (TB 5)	Together, these points clear heat in the upper burner and especially in the heart.
Xue Hai (Sp 10) *Nei Ting* (St 44)	Together, these points clear heat and cool the blood.
San Yin Jiao (Sp 6)	Enriches yin to enhance cooling the blood

Chinese medicinal formula: Modified *Dao Chi San* (Abduct the Red Decoction) plus *Huang Lian Jie Du Tang* (Coptis Resolve Toxins Decoction)

Ingredients: Wine stir-fried Rhizoma Coptidis Chinensis (*Huang Lian*), 6g, wine stir-fried Radix Scutellariae Baicalensis (*Huang Qin*), 6g, uncooked Cortex Phellodendri (*Huang Bai*), 6g, uncooked Fructus Gardeniae Jasminoidis (*Zhi Zi*), 9g, uncooked Radix Rehmanniae (*Sheng Di*), 9g,

Herba Lophatheri Gracilis (*Dan Zhu Ye*), 3g, Caulis Akebiae (*Mu Tong*), 6g, Rhizoma Imperatae Cylindricae (*Bai Mao Gen*), 12g, Flos Immaturus Sophorae Japonicae (*Huai Hua Mi*), 12g, Nodus Rhizomatis Nelumbinis Nuciferae (*Ou Jie*), 12g, Radix Glycyrrhizae (*Gan Cao*), 3g

Additions & subtractions: If there is severe bleeding, add Cacumen Biotae Orientalis (*Ce Bai Ye*), 9g, and Herba Agrimoniae Pilosae (*Xian He Cao*), 9g.

2. Liver fire harassing above

Symptoms: Persistent bleeding from the tongue, a hard, swollen tongue with yellow fur and red crimson tongue edges, red face and eyes, a bitter taste in the mouth, irascibility, headache, dizziness, vertigo, tinnitus, deafness, burning pain in the lateral costal region, short voidings of yellow, dark-colored urine, constipation, and a wiry, rapid pulse

Therapeutic principles: Clear the liver and drain fire, cool the blood and stop bleeding

Acupuncture & moxibustion:

Xing Jian (Liv 2)	Together, these points clear the liver, drain fire,
Qi Men (Liv 14)	and stop bleeding.
Feng Chi (GB 20)	

Qu Quan (Liv 8)	Enriches yin to help downbear fire
Yong Quan (Ki 1)	Together, these points lead fire downward and
Da Dun (Liv 1)	drain fire to cool the blood when needled with
Xue Hai (Sp 10)	draining method.

Chinese medicinal formula: Modified *Dang Gui Long Hui Wan* (Dang Gui & Aloe Pills)

Ingredients: Uncooked Radix Angelicae Sinensis (*Dang Gui*), 9g, Radix Gentianae Scabrae (*Long Dan Cao*), 9g, Fructus Gardeniae Jasminoidis (*Zhi Zi*), 6g, wine stir-fried Radix Scutellariae Baicalensis (*Huang Qin*), 6g, wine stir-fried Rhizoma Coptidis Chinensis (*Huang Lian*), 6g, uncooked Cortex Phellodendri (*Huang Bai*), 6g, uncooked Radix Et Rhizoma Rhei (*Da Huang*), 6g, Radix Auklandiae Lappae (*Mu Xiang*), 3g, Cacumen Biotae Orientalis (*Ce Bai Ye*), 9g, Rhizoma Imperatae Cylindricae (*Bai Mao Gen*), 12g, Radix Glycyrrhizae (*Gan Cao*), 6g

3. Yin vacuity fire flaring upward

Symptoms: Oozing of blood from the tongue which is small in amount, red cheekbones, dizziness, flowery (*i.e.*, blurred) vision, dry mouth and throat, emaciation, tinnitus, reduced sleep, impaired memory, pain and weakness of the low back and knees, vexatious heat in the five hearts, tidal fever, night sweats, loose teeth, a thin, red tongue with reduced fur, and a fine, rapid pulse

Therapeutic principles: Enrich yin, downbear fire, and stop bleeding

Acupuncture & moxibustion:

Gan Shu (Bl 18)	Together, these points enrich and nourish yin and
Shen Shu (Bl 23)	blood, while *Ge Shu* also stops bleeding.
Pi Shu (Bl 20)	
Ge Shu (Bl 17)	

Fu Liu (Ki 7)	Together, these points enrich yin and downbear
Yong Quan (KI 1)	fire to stop bleeding.

Chinese medicinal formula: Modified *Zhi Bai Di Huang Wan* (Anemarrhena & Phellodendron Rehmannia Pills)

Ingredients: Prepared Radix Rehmanniae (*Shu Di*), 18g, uncooked Radix Dioscoreae Oppositae (*Shan Yao*), 9g, steamed Fructus Corni Officinalis (*Shan Zhu Yu*), 9g, Sclerotium Poriae Cocos (*Fu Ling*), 6g, salt mix-fried Rhizoma Alismatis (*Ze Xie*), 6g, Cortex Radicis Moutan (*Dan Pi*), 12g, salt mix-fried Rhizoma Anemarrhenae Asphodeloidis (*Zhi Mu*), 9g, salt mix-fried Cortex Phellodendri (*Huang Bai*), 9g, salt stir-fried Radix Achyranthis Bidentatae (*Niu Xi*), 9g, Flos Immaturus Sophorae Japonicae (*Huai Hua Mi*), 9g, Cacumen Biotae Orientalis (*Ce Bai Ye*), 9g

4. Spleen failing to contain the blood

Symptoms: Oozing blood from the tongue which is pale in color and thin in consistency, a lusterless facial complexion, pale lips and nails, reduced food intake, fatigue, spontaneous perspiration, shortage of qi, fatigued spirit with disinclination to speak, a fat, tender, pale tongue with white fur, and a fine, forceless pulse

Therapeutic principles: Boost the qi and contain the blood

Acupuncture & moxibustion:

Pi Shu (Bl 20)	Together, these points fortify the spleen, boost the
Ge Shu (Bl 17)	qi, and contain the blood when needled with
Zu San Li (St 36)	supplementing method.

Guan Yuan (CV 4)	Together, when moxaed, these points supplement
Qi Hai (CV 6)	the qi to support the center qi.

Chinese medicinal formula: Modified *Gui Pi Tang* (Return the Spleen Decoction)

Ingredients: Honey stir-fried Radix Astragali Membranacei (*Huang Qi*), 12g, bran stir-fried Rhizoma Atractylodis Macrocephalae (*Bai Zhu*), 9g, stir-fried Radix Angelicae Sinensis (*Dang Gui*), 9g, Arillus Euphoriae

Longanae (*Long Yan Rou*), 6g, Sclerotium Poriae Cocos (*Fu Ling*), 9g, Radix Auklandiae Lappae (*Mu Xiang*), 3g, mix-fried Radix Glycyrrhizae (*Zhi Gan Cao*), 6g, Radix Codonopsitis Pilosulae (*Dang Shen*), 12g, stir-fried Semen Zizyphi Spinosae (*Suan Zao Ren*), 6g, Pollen Typhae (*Pu Huang*), 9g

30
Tongue Sores (*She Chuang*)

This refers to ulceration and inflammation of the surface of the tongue which is slow to heal.

Disease causes, disease mechanisms:

I. Intense heart fire

Intense heart fire is mainly due to excesses of the five affects, such as over-thinking, that transform fire. "The heart opens into the tongue" and the diverging network vessels of the heart connect with the root of the tongue. Therefore, if heart fire flames upward along these channels to the tongue, it may burn and damage the network vessels in the tongue, leading to tongue sores.

2. Stomach fire fuming & steaming

Stomach fire may arise from addiction to alcohol or rich flavoured, spicy, and/or fried food that engenders heat. If heat brews and accumulates in the stomach duct, it will fume, steam, and then flame upward since, "Fire by nature flames upward." Upflaming, this heat may burn and damage the network vessels in the tongue, leading to tongue sores.

3. Central qi vacuity

Central qi vacuity may be the result of dietary irregularities, taxation, and/or enduring disease. The central qi is responsible for upbearing the clear yang. If it becomes vacuous, the center qi may fail to do that. Consequently, the clear yang will fail to bear upward and may become depressed, giving rise to the formation of heat internally. If this heat steams upward, there may be tongue sores.

4. Blood vacuity

Blood vacuity may arise from over thinking, massive loss of the blood, or spleen vacuity. Blood vacuity may engender dryness and, in turn, this dryness can transform heat. If dry heat flames upward, there may be tongue sores.

5. Kidney vacuity

Kidney vacuity may be from enduring disease, taxation, and/or unrestrained sexual activity. If kidney yin is vacuous, yang will become hyperactive, giving rise to yin vacuity fire. If kidney yang is vacuous, there will be failure of the kidney storing, resulting in rootless, upwardly floating fire. If either yin vacuity fire or floating fire goes upward to the tongue along the channels, tongue sores may occur.

Treatment based on pattern discrimination:

I. Intense heart fire

Symptoms: A painful, bright red surface to the eruption on the tongue, especially on the tongue tip, accompanied by a red face, thirst, vexatious heat in the chest, disquieted sleep at night, astringent voidings of dark-colored urine, a red tongue or crimson red tongue tip, and a rapid pulse or rapid, big pulse at the *cun* portion on the left side.

Therapeutic principles: Clear the heart and drain fire

Acupuncture & moxibustion:

Jin Jin (M-HN-20b)   Clears heat in the local area when pricked to
Yu Ye (M-HN-20a)   bleed

| Guan Chong (TB 1) | Together, these points clear heat in the upper |
| Wai Guan (TB 5) | burner and especially in the heart. |

| Lao Gong (Per 8) | Together, these points clear the heart and drain |
| Yong Quan (Ki 1) | fire. *Yong Quan* also leads fire downward. |

Chinese medicinal formula: Modified *Dao Chi San* (Abduct the Red Decoction)

Ingredients: Uncooked Radix Rehmanniae (*Sheng Di*), 12g, Caulis Akebiae (*Mu Tong*), 6g, Radix Tenuis Glycyrrhizae (*Gan Cao Shao*), 9g, Herba Lophatheri Gracilis (*Dan Zhu Ye*), 9g, Rhizoma Coptidis Chinensis (*Huang Lian*), 6g, stir-fried Fructus Gardeniae Jasminoidis (*Zhi Zi*), 9g, Radix Scrophulariae Ningpoensis (*Xuan Shen*), 6g, stir-fried till scorched Fructus Meliae Toosendan (*Chuan Lian Zi*), 9g

2. Stomach fire fuming & steaming

Symptoms: A relatively larger opening to the eruption on the tongue accompanied by bad breath, thirst with a liking for chilled drinks, easy hungering with clamoring stomach, constipation, a red tongue with yellow, dry or yellow, thick fur, and a slippery, rapid pulse

Therapeutic principles: Clear heat and resolve toxins, drain fire and free the stools

Acupuncture & moxibustion:

| Jin Jin (M-HN-20b) | Clears heat in the local area when pricked to bleed |
| Yu Ye (M-HN-20a) | |

| Shi Xuan (M-UE-1) | Drains fire and resolves toxins when pricked to bleed |

He Gu (LI 4)	Together, these points clear heat and free the
Tian Shu (St 25)	stools.
Shang Ju Xu (St 37)	

Chinese medicinal formula: Modified *Liang Ge San* (Cool the Diaphragm Powder)

Ingredients: Fructus Forsythiae Suspensae (*Lian Qiao*), 15g, uncooked Radix Et Rhizoma Rhei (*Da Huang*), 9g, Mirabilitum (*Mang Xiao*), 9g, Fructus Gardeniae Jasminoidis (*Zhi Zi*), 9g, Radix Scutellariae Baicalensis (*Huang Qin*), 9g, Herba Menthae Haplocalysis (*Bo He*), 6g, Radix Glycyrrhizae (*Gan Cao*), 9g, wine stir-fried Rhizoma Coptidis Chinensis (*Huang Lian*), 6g

3. Central qi vacuity

Symptoms: Obstinate sores on the tongue with the opening of the sore falling downward accompanied by fatigued limbs, shortage of qi with disinclination to speak, low fever, a pale tongue with thin, white fur, and a soft, forceless or vacuous, big, rapid pulse

Therapeutic principles: Supplement the center and boost the qi

Acupuncture & moxibustion:

Lian Quan (CV 23)	Quickens the channel qi in the local area
Bai Hui (GV 20)	Upbears clear yang when moxaed on the handle of the needle
Zu San Li (St 36)	Together, these points supplement the center and
He Gu (LI 4)	boost the qi when needled with supplementing method.

Chinese medicinal formula: Modified *Bu Zhong Yi Qi Tang* (Supplement the Center & Boost the Qi Decoction)

Ingredients: Honey stir-fried Radix Astragali Membranacei (*Huang Qi*), 12g, mix-fried Radix Glycyrrhizae (*Zhi Gan Cao*), 6g, honey stir-fried Radix Codonopsitis Pilosulae (*Dang Shen*), 9g, bran stir-fried Rhizoma Atractylodis Macrocephalae (*Bai Zhu*), 9g, stir-fried Radix Angelicae Sinensis (*Dang Gui*), 9g, stir-fried Pericarpium Citri Reticulatae (*Chen Pi*), 6g, honey mix-fried Rhizoma Cimicifugae (*Sheng Ma*), 3g, stir-fried Radix Bupleuri (*Chai Hu*), 3g, Sclerotium Poriae Cocos (*Fu Ling*), 9g, Tuber Ophiopogonis Japonici (*Mai Men Dong*), 9g, Fructus Schisandrae Chinensis (*Wu Wei Zi*), 9g

4. Blood vacuity

Symptoms: Obstinate sores on the tongue accompanied by dry mouth with no desire to drink, dizziness, flowery (*i.e.,* blurred) vision, disturbed sleep, a sensation of heat in the hands and feet, fatigue and lack of strength, inhibited throat, a pale red tongue with thin, white fur or no fur, and a fine, rapid or vacuous, weak pulse

Therapeutic principles: Nourish the blood and clear dry heat

Acupuncture & moxibustion:

Lian Quan (CV 23)	Engenders fluids and clears heat in the local area
Zu San Li (St 36) *San Yin Jiao* (Sp 6)	Together, these points fortify the spleen and stomach to enhance the source of engendering and transforming. In addition, *San Yin Jiao* nourishes yin to clear dry heat.
Pi Shu (Bl 20) *Wei Shu* (Bl 21)	Together, these points nourish the blood.

Chinese medicinal formula: Modified *Si Wu Tang* (Four Ingredients Decoction)

Ingredients: Prepared Radix Rehmanniae (*Shu Di*), 12g, uncooked Radix Rehmanniae (*Sheng Di*), 9g, uncooked Radix Albus Paeoniae Lactiflorae (*Bai Shao*), 12g, wine mix-fried Radix Angelicae Sinensis (*Dang Gui*), 9g, wine mix-fried Radix Ligustici Wallichii (*Chuan Xiong*), 6g, Rhizoma Anemarrhenae Asphodeloidis (*Zhi Mu*), 6g, Cortex Phellodendri (*Huang Bai*), 6g, Cortex Radicis Moutan (*Dan Pi*), 9g, Tuber Ophiopogonis Japonici (*Mai Men Dong*), 9g, Fructus Schisandrae Chinensis (*Wu Wei Zi*), 9g

5. Kidney yin vacuity

Symptoms: Obstinate, red sores on the tongue accompanied by sore throat, dry mouth, tinnitus, vertigo, seminal emission, low backache which is worse in the late afternoon, a red, dry tongue, and a fine, rapid pulse

Therapeutic principles: Enrich yin and downbear fire

Acupuncture & moxibustion:

Lian Quan (CV 23) *Tong Li* (Ht 5)	Together, these points engender fluids. In addition, *Tong Li* downbears heart fire.
San Yin Jiao (Sp 6) *Tai Xi* (Ki 3) *Yong Quan* (Ki 1)[9]	Together, these points enrich yin and downbear fire.

Chinese medicinal formula: Modified *Zhi Bai Di Huang Wan* (Anemarrhena & Phellodendron Rehmannia Pills)

---

[9] Because *Yong Quan* can be a painful point to needle, instead one can apply a paste to this point. This paste is made from mixing powdered Cortex Cinnamomi Cassiae (*Rou Gui*) with vinegar. Hold in place with an adhesive plaster.

Ingredients: Prepared Radix Rehmanniae (*Shu Di*), 18g, uncooked Radix Dioscoreae Oppositae (*Shan Yao*), 9g, steamed Fructus Corni Officinalis (*Shan Zhu Yu*), 9g, Sclerotium Poriae Cocos (*Fu Ling*), 6g, salt mix-fried Rhizoma Alismatis (*Ze Xie*), 6g, Cortex Radicis Moutan (*Dan Pi*), 12g, salt mix-fried Rhizoma Anemarrhenae Asphodeloidis (*Zhi Mu*), 9g, salt mix-fried Cortex Phellodendri (*Huang Bai*), 9g, salt stir-fried Radix Achyranthis Bidentatae (*Niu Xi*), 9g, Radix Scrophulariae Ningpoensis (*Xuan Shen*), 9g

6. Kidney yang vacuity

Symptoms: Obstinate sores on the tongue accompanied by a pale white facial complexion, chilled limbs, loose stools, impotence, frequent urination, low back and knee pain and weakness, a pale tongue with thin, white fur, and a deep, slow pulse

Therapeutic principles: Warm and supplement the kidneys, contain floating fire

Acupuncture & moxibustion:

Lian Quan (CV 23)	Quickens the network vessels
Bai Hui (GB 20)	When moxaed, upbears yang
Guan Yuan Shu (Bl 26) *Qi Hai Shu* (Bl 24) *Ming Men* (GV 4)	Together, when moxaed, these points warm and supplement kidney yang to lead floating fire back to its lower source.

Mix smashed Fructus Evodiae Rutecarpae (*Wu Zhu Yu*) with vinegar and then apply this mixture as a compress on *Yong Quan* (Ki 1) during night.

Chinese medicinal formula: *Shen Qi Wan* (Kidney Qi Pills)

Ingredients: Prepared Radix Rehmanniae (*Shu Di*), 18g, stir-fried Radix Dioscoreae Oppositae (*Shan Yao*), 12g, steamed Fructus Corni Officinalis

(*Shan Zhu Yu*), 12g, salt mix-fried Rhizoma Alismatis (*Ze Xie*), 9g, Sclerotium Poriae Cocos (*Fu Ling*), 9g, Cortex Radicis Moutan (*Dan Pi*), 9g, Cortex Cinnamomi Cassiae (*Rou Gui*), 3g, bland Radix Lateralis Praeparatus Aconiti Carmichaeli (*Fu Zi*), 6g

Note: The Chinese disease category of sores on the tongue covers relatively wide ground, from pediatric thrush to adult aphthous stomatitis. When such sores are episodic, they are more often associated with replete patterns such as heart or liver heat. When they are recurrent or recalcitrant to treatment, they are usually a combination of righteous vacuity mixed with some sort of evil heat. Aphthous stomatitis is a fungal or yeast condition at least locally. However, proliferation of yeast in an otherwise immune compromised patient is a potential danger sign of a deteriorating condition. Persons with compromised immune systems include those with chronic allergies, autoimmune diseases, immune deficiency conditions (such as AIDS & CFIDS), and those with serious, life-threatening diseases such as cancer. When patients with such conditions manifest sores on the tongue, their diets must immediately be corrected to eliminate foods which either damage the spleen or give rise to dampness and heat, while initiating internal treatment to rectify their pattern. If one overlooks the diet, Chinese medicinals alone will either not achieve a satisfactory effect or the condition will quickly relapse.

31
Worrying Tongue (*Nong She*)

Worrying tongue refers to repeatedly licking the lips and corners of the mouth or restlessly sticking the tip of the tongue out and then quickly withdrawing it.

Disease causes, disease mechanisms:

I. Replete heat in the heart & spleen

Such replete heat may be due to excesses of the five affects or addiction to alcohol and spicy, greasy food. The heart and spleen channels both connect with the tongue. If heat remains and brews in the heart and spleen channels, it may go upward and disquiet the tongue since heat is a yang evil and the nature of yang is to move. Therefore, there is worrying tongue.

2. Vacuous heat in the spleen & kidneys

In late stage febrile disease, spleen and kidney yin have often been consumed and damaged even though evils have been expelled. In addition, some enduring diseases may also consume spleen and kidney yin. Vacuous heat is engendered when yin is vacuous. If there is vacuity heat, first the tongue will be disquieted, and secondly, yin fluids will be burnt and become damaged. This then leads to less nourishment to the sinews of the tongue and thus a tense tongue. In order to relax such a tense tongue, the patient tends to lick their lips and the corners of their mouth. Therefore, there is worrying tongue.

3. Phlegm confounding the portals of the heart

Worrying tongue can also be one of the symptoms of apoplexy associated with a combination of wind and phlegm blocking the portals of the heart. This wind mainly comes from liver-kidney yin vacuity rendering yang unchecked or from excesses of the five affects transforming into fire and then engendering wind. The phlegm may be constitutional or may be due to dietary irregularities that damage the spleen. Thus the spleen fails to transform dampness and this dampness accumulates and eventually is congealed into phlegm. It is also possible for heat to burn liquids into phlegm. If wind drafts this phlegm upward resulting in blockage of the root of the tongue or clouds the clear portals, there will be stiff tongue if phlegm predominates and a worrying tongue if wind predominates. A worrying tongue due to wind phlegm obstruction is usually associated with the sequelae of windstroke or apoplexy or may be associated with an epileptic seizure.

Treatment based on pattern discrimination:

I. Replete heat in the heart & spleen

Symptoms: Quickly sticking the tongue in and out, fever, a red face, occasional vexation and agitation, thirst and a liking for chilled drinks, dry lips and mouth, sores on the mouth and tongue, constipation or foul defecation, a red tongue with yellow, dry fur, and a wiry, rapid, or surging, rapid pulse

Therapeutic principles: Clear heat and drain fire

Acupuncture & moxibustion:

Shao Hai (Ht 3)   Clears the heart and quiets the spirit

Wen Liu (Ll 7)   Together, these points drain heat in the spleen and
Hua Rou Men (St 24)   stomach.
Yin Bai (Sp 1)

Additions & subtractions: For bad breath, add *Da Ling* (Per 7). For a bitter taste in the mouth, add *Yang Ling Quan* (GB 34).

Chinese medicinal formula: Modified *Qing Wei San* (Clear Stomach Powder)

Ingredients: Wine stir-fried Rhizoma Coptidis Chinensis (*Huang Lian*), 6g, uncooked Radix Rehmanniae (*Sheng Di*), 15g, uncooked Radix Angelicae Sinensis (*Dang Gui*), 9g, Cortex Radicis Moutan (*Dan Pi*), 6g, uncooked Rhizoma Cimicifugae (*Sheng Ma*), 6g, Radix Glycyrrhizae (*Gan Cao*), 6g, Tuber Ophiopogonis Japonici (*Mai Men Dong*), 6g, Plumula Nelumbinis Nuciferae (*Lian Xin*), 3g

Additions & subtractions: If there is constipation, add uncooked Radix Et Rhizoma Rhei (*Da Huang*), 9g, and Mirabilitum (*Mang Xiao*), 6g. If heat damages the fluids, add uncooked Gypsum Fibrosum (*Shi Gao*), 15g, and uncooked Radix Rehmanniae (*Sheng Di*), 9g.

2. Vacuous heat in the spleen & kidneys

Symptoms: Sticking out the tongue from time to time and keeping the tongue out for a relatively longer time, drooling from the corners of the mouth, vexatious heat in the five hearts, thirst with a desire to drink, a red tongue with reduced fur, and a fine, rapid pulse

Therapeutic principles: Fortify the spleen and boost the kidneys, enrich yin and clear heat

Acupuncture & moxibustion:

Da Du (Sp 2)	Together, these points fortify the spleen. In
Zu San Li (St 36)	addition, *Da Du* clears heat in the spleen.
Fu Liu (Ki 7)	Together, these points enrich yin and boost the
Tai Xi (Ki 3)	kidneys. *Fu Liu* also clears heat in the kidneys.

Chinese medicinal formula: Modified *Zhi Bai Di Huang Wan* (Anemarrhena & Phellodendron Rehmannia Pills)

Ingredients: Prepared Radix Rehmanniae (*Shu Di*), 18g, uncooked Radix Dioscoreae Oppositae (*Shan Yao*), 9g, steamed Fructus Corni Officinalis (*Shan Zhu Yu*), 9g, Sclerotium Poriae Cocos (*Fu Ling*), 6g, salt mix-fried Rhizoma Alismatis (*Ze Xie*), 6g, Cortex Radicis Moutan (*Dan Pi*), 12g, salt mix-fried Rhizoma Anemarrhenae Asphodeloidis (*Zhi Mu*), 9g, salt mix-fried Cortex Phellodendri (*Huang Bai*), 9g, uncooked Radix Codonopsitis Pilosulae (*Dang Shen*), 9g, Rhizoma Atractylodis Macrocephalae (*Bai Zhu*), 6g, mix-fried Radix Glycyrrhizae (*Zhi Gan Cao*), 6g

32
Protracted Tongue (*She Zong*)

Protracted tongue refers to an elongated, loosened tongue where the patient sticks their tongue out but then has difficulty withdrawing it back into their mouth. In some cases, the tongue cannot be retracted. In English, this can be called a lolling tongue, whereas the Chinese implies something that is both elongated and which has been released or set loose. This condition is often accompanied by drooling.

Disease causes, disease mechanisms:

1. Intense heart fire

Intense heart fire may arise due to excesses of the five affects, for example, over-thinking consuming heart yin and blood leading to heat exuberance of the heart. "The heart opens into the tongue." If intense heart fire flames upward to the tongue along the channel, it may render the tongue slack or loose and this may lead to a protracted tongue. If heat damages the fluids in the tongue, the tongue will protract due to hypertonicity. If heat is coupled with phlegm, the tongue will be distended and full.

2. Liver qi depression & binding

Liver qi depression and binding mainly develops from emotional disturbances like frustration, anger, and depression. If the depressed liver qi bursts, attacks upward, and then congests in the tongue, the qi mechanism in the tongue will be inhibited, leading to protracted tongue.

3. Qi vacuity

Qi vacuity may be due to enduring disease, taxation, and/or spleen vacuity. Qi is supposed to govern securing and containment. If the qi is vacuous, securing and containment may fail, and, therefore, there may be a protracted tongue.

Treatment based on pattern discrimination:

I. Intense heart fire

Symptoms: A red, tense, dry, protracted tongue that is difficult to withdraw or even cannot be drawn back into the mouth, a red face, vexation, thirst, dark-colored urine, and a rapid, forceful pulse. When heat is coupled with phlegm, the tongue is fat and distended as well.

Therapeutic principles: Clear the heart and drain fire

Acupuncture & moxibustion:

Shao Chong (Ht 9)	Together, these points clear heat in the heart,
Shen Men (Ht 7)	while *Shen Men* also nourishes heart yin.
Dui Duan (GV 27)	Together, these points drain fire, while *Yong Quan*
Yong Quan (Ki 1)	also leads heat downward.

Additions & subtractions: For signs of phlegm, add *Feng Long* (St 40). Use a filiform needle and prick the tip of the tongue if the tongue cannot be withdrawn.

Chinese medicinal formula: Modified *Xie Xin Tang* (Drain the Heart Decoction)

Ingredients: Wine stir-fried Radix Scutellariae Baicalensis (*Huang Qin*), 9g, wine stir-fried Rhizoma Coptidis Chinensis (*Huang Lian*), 6g, uncooked Radix Et Rhizoma Rhei (*Da Huang*), 6-9g, Rhizoma

Anemarrhenae Asphodeloidis (*Zhi Mu*), 9g, Folium Bambusae (*Zhu Ye*), 9g, Rhizoma Acori Graminei (*Shi Chang Pu*), 9g, Plumula Nelumbinis Nuciferae (*Lian Xin*), 3g

Additions & subtractions: If there is phlegm, subtract Plumula Nelumbinis Nuciferae (*Lian Xin*) and add lime-processed Rhizoma Pinelliae Ternatae (*Ban Xia*), 9g, Sclerotium Poriae Cocos (*Fu Ling*), 9g, Pericarpium Citri Reticulatae (*Chen Pi*), 6g, bile-processed Rhizoma Arisaematis (*Dan Nan Xing*), 9g, and Bombyx Batryticatus (*Jiang Can*), 9g.

2. Liver qi depression & binding

Symptoms: A protracted tongue which can be withdrawn, a recent history of emotional disturbance, but no other symptoms except possible oppression and distention in the chest and lateral costal region, depression, frequent sighing, poor appetite, and a wiry pulse

Therapeutic principles: Course the liver and resolve depression

Acupuncture & moxibustion:

Lian Quan (CV 23)	Frees the flow of the network vessels in the tongue
Qi Men (Liv 14) *Tai Chong* (Liv 3)	Together, these points course the liver and resolve depression.

Chinese medicinal formula: *Xiao Yao San* (Rambling Powder)

Ingredients: Radix Bupleuri (*Chai Hu*), 6g, bran stir-fried Rhizoma Atractylodis Macrocephalae (*Bai Zhu*), 9g, uncooked Radix Albus Paeoniae Lactiflorae (*Bai Shao*), 9g, wine mix-fried Radix Angelicae Sinensis (*Dang Gui*), 9g, Sclerotium Poriae Cocos (*Fu Ling*), 6g, Herba Menthae Haplocalysis (*Bo He*), 3g, mix-fried Radix Glycyrrhizae (*Zhi Gan Cao*), 3g, uncooked Rhizoma Zingiberis (*Sheng Jiang*), 3g

Additions & subtractions: If liver depression transforms into heat, add uncooked Radix Scutellariae Baicalensis (*Huang Qin*), 9g, uncooked Fructus Gardeniae Jasminoidis (*Zhi Zi*), 9g, and Cortex Radicis Moutan (*Dan Pi*), 9g.

3. Qi vacuity

Symptoms: A protracted, numb, tender, soft tongue which is too slack to withdraw accompanied by fatigue and lack of strength, reduced qi with disinclination to speak, spontaneous sweating, thin, white tongue fur, and a vacuous, weak pulse

Therapeutic principles: Supplement the center and boost the qi

Acupuncture & moxibustion:

Lian Quan (CV 23)	Quickens the channel qi in the local area
He Gu (LI 4)	Together, these points supplement the center and
Zu San Li (St 36)	boost the qi.
Shan Zhong (CV 17)	

Chinese medicinal formula: *Bu Zhong Yi Qi Tang* (Supplement the Center & Boost the Qi Decoction)

Ingredients: Honey stir-fried Radix Astragali Membranacei (*Huang Qi*), 12g, mix-fried Radix Glycyrrhizae (*Zhi Gan Cao*), 6g, honey stir-fried Radix Codonopsitis Pilosulae (*Dang Shen*), 9g, bran stir-fried Rhizoma Atractylodis Macrocephalae (*Bai Zhu*), 9g, stir-fried Radix Angelicae Sinensis (*Dang Gui*), 9g, stir-fried Pericarpium Citri Reticulatae (*Chen Pi*), 6g, honey mix-fried Rhizoma Cimicifugae (*Sheng Ma*), 3g, stir-fried Radix Bupleuri (*Chai Hu*), 3g

33
Loosening of the Teeth (*Ya Chi Song Dong*)

Loosening of the teeth refers to teeth which are not firm and can be easily shaken.

Disease causes, disease mechanisms:

The hand *yang ming* channel enters the lower teeth and the foot *yang ming* channel enters the upper, while the teeth are the surplus of the bone which is governed by the kidneys. Therefore, loosening of the teeth is often associated with the *yang ming* and kidneys.

I. Heat congesting in the *yang ming*

This heat is often due to addiction to alcohol, spicy, and/or rich-flavoured food which may engender heat. Accumulating and congesting in the stomach duct, the heat may steam and then go upward to the gums along the channel, burning and putrefying the flesh of the gums. If the gums that support and fasten the teeth become putrefied, the root part of the teeth will be exposed and thus become loose.

2. Kidney qi vacuity

Kidney qi vacuity may be due to constitutional kidney insufficiency, aging, or enduring disease. Kidney qi is responsible for securing. If it becomes vacuous, it cannot secure the teeth and, therefore, the teeth will become loose.

3. Kidney yin vacuity

Kidney yin vacuity mainly arises from unrestrained sexual activity, enduring seminal emission, or aging leading to insufficiency of kidney essence. Kidney essence is responsible for engendering the marrow, and the marrow is supposed to engender the bone. The teeth are the surplus of the bones and thus need nourishment from the marrow. If kidney yin becomes vacuous, the teeth cannot get sufficient nourishment and hence become loose.

Treatment based on pattern discrimination:

I. Heat congesting in the *yang ming*

Symptoms: Loose teeth accompanied by red, swollen gums, possible gaping gums, bad breath, constipation, thirst and a liking for chilled drinks, a red tongue with yellow, slimy, dryish fur, and a slippery, rapid pulse

Therapeutic principles: Clear the stomach and secure the teeth

Acupuncture & moxibustion:

He Gu (LI 4) *Er Jian* (LI 2)	Together, these points clear heat in the *yang ming*.
Ren Zhong (GV 26)	An intersection point of the governing vessel, stomach, and spleen channels which drains heat to secure the teeth
Di Cang (St 4) *Nei Ting* (St 44)	Together, these points clear the stomach to secure the teeth.

Chinese medicinal formula: Modified *Qing Wei San* (Clear Stomach Powder)

Ingredients: Uncooked Gypsum Fibrosum (*Shi Gao*), 20g, wine stir-fried Rhizoma Coptidis Chinensis (*Huang Lian*), 6g, uncooked Radix Rehmanniae (*Sheng Di*), 20g, uncooked Radix Angelicae Sinensis (*Dang Gui*), 9g, Cortex Radicis Moutan (*Dan Pi*), 9g, uncooked Rhizoma Cimicifugae (*Sheng Ma*), 3g, Radix Glycyrrhizae (*Gan Cao*), 3g, Fructus Gardeniae Jasminoidis (*Zhi Zi*), 9g, uncooked Radix Et Rhizoma Rhei (*Da Huang*), 6g

2. Kidney qi vacuity

Symptoms: Loose teeth or even falling of the teeth mainly encountered in the elderly patients, difficulty chewing accompanied by pain and weakness of the low back and knees, fatigued spirit, dizziness, vertigo, reduced auditory acuity, frequent urination at night, dribbling voidings of clear urine, loose stools, a pale, tender, moist tongue with white fur, and a deep, fine pulse, weak at the *chi* position

Therapeutic principles: Supplement the kidneys and boost the qi

Acupuncture & moxibustion:

Guan Yuan (CV 4) *Qi Hai* (CV 6) *Ming Men* (GV 4)	Together, these points boost kidney qi.
Shen Shu (Bl 23) *Zhi Shi* (Bl 52)	Together, these points supplement the essence to transform qi.

Chinese medicinal formula: Modified *Huan Shao Dan* (Give Back [What Has] Disappeared Elixir)

Ingredients: Prepared Radix Rehmanniae (*Shu Di*), 18g, stir-fried Radix Dioscoreae Oppositae (*Shan Yao*), 9g, steamed Fructus Corni Officinalis (*Shan Zhu Yu*), 9g, salt stir-fried Radix Achyranthis Bidentatae (*Niu Xi*), 9g, Fructus Lycii Chinensis (*Gou Qi*), 9g, Sclerotium Poriae Cocos (*Fu Ling*), 9g, salt stir-fried Cortex Eucommiae Ulmoidis (*Du Zhong*), 9g, Fructus Schisandrae Chinensis (*Wu Wei Zi*), 9g, Rhizoma Drynariae (*Gu Sui Bu*), 9g, Cornu Parvum Cervi (*Lu Rong*), 1g (powdered), Herba Cistanchis Deserticolae (*Rou Cong Rong*), 9g, Rhizoma Acori Graminei (*Shi Chang Pu*), 6g, Fructus Zizyphi Jujubae (*Da Zao*), 3 pieces

3. Kidney yin vacuity

Symptoms: Loose teeth followed by gaping gums and accompanied by low backache, dry mouth, dizziness, tinnitus, hair loss, tidal fever, night sweats, a thin, red tongue with thin, yellow or reduced fur, and a fine, rapid pulse

Therapeutic principles: Enrich yin and downbear fire to secure the teeth

Acupuncture & moxibustion:

Tai Xi (Ki 3) *Fu Liu* (Ki 7)	Together, these points enrich yin and downbear fire.
Xuan Zhong (GB 39) *Shen Shu* (Bl 23)	The meeting point of the marrow, together with *Shen Shu*, boosts the kidneys to secure the teeth.

Chinese medicinal formula: Modified *Liu Wei Di Huang Wan* (Six Flavors Rehmannia Pills)

Ingredients: Prepared Radix Rehmanniae (*Shu Di*), 24g, steamed Fructus Corni Officinalis (*Shan Zhu Yu*), 12g, stir-fried Radix Dioscoreae Oppositae (*Shan Yao*), 12g, Sclerotium Poriae Cocos (*Fu Ling*), 6g, Cortex Radicis Moutan (*Dan Pi*), 6g, Rhizoma Alismatis (*Ze Xie*), 6g,

Rhizoma Drynariae (*Gu Sui Bu*), 9g, salt stir-fried Radix Achyranthis Bidentatae (*Niu Xi*), 9g

Additions & subtractions: If vacuity heat signs are severe, add salt mix-fried Cortex Phellodendri (*Huang Bai*), 9g, and salt mix-fried Rhizoma Anemarrhenae Asphodeloidis (*Zhi Mu*), 9g.

34
Blackening of the Teeth (*Ya Chi Jiao Hei*)

Blackening of the teeth refers to a condition where the teeth become dry, yellowish, and black. This is different from the blackish tartar that can be removed by scrapping.

Disease causes, disease mechanisms:

Blackening of the teeth is an important diagnostic sign in warm disease showing that heat evils have entered the lower burner.

I. Exuberant heat in the lower burner

In late stage warm disease, evils often enter the lower burner and become even more difficult to resolve. Heat evils always consume fluids. If heat in the lower burner consumes, damages, and exhausts the fluids, the teeth will get less moistening and nourishment, thus leading to blackening of the teeth.

2. Kidney heat & stomach dryness

In late stage warm disease, stomach fluids and kidney fluids often become exhausted. The stomach channel enters the teeth, while the teeth are the surplus of the bones which are governed by the kidneys. With exhaustion of fluids, the teeth cannot get sufficient moisture and nourishment, thus leading to blackening of the teeth.

Treatment based on pattern discrimination:

I. Exuberant heat in the lower burner

Symptoms: Blackening of the teeth with no grime, dry mouth and tongue, wriggling of the fingers (*i.e.*, carpalpholgia), and a deep, rapid pulse

Therapeutic principles: Foster yin and engender fluids

Acupuncture & moxibustion:

Fu Liu (Ki 7)	Together, these points nourish yin and engender
Tai Xi (Ki 3)	fluids. *Fu Liu* also clears heat in the lower burner.
San Yin Jiao (Sp 6)	

Shen Shu (Bl 23)	Together, these points enrich the kidneys to foster
Zhi Shi (Bl 52)	yin.

Chinese medicinal formula: *Er Jia Fu Mai Tang* (Two Shells Restore the Pulse Decoction)

Ingredients: Uncooked Concha Ostreae (*Mu Li*), 15g, uncooked Carapax Amydae Sinensis (*Bie Jia*), 15g, uncooked Radix Rehmanniae (*Sheng Di*), 15g, uncooked Radix Albus Paeoniae Lactiflorae (*Bai Shao*), 15g, Tuber Ophiopogonis Japonici (*Mai Men Dong*), 9g, Gelatinum Corii Asini (*E Jiao*), 6g, Semen Cannabis Sativae (*Huo Ma Ren*), 6g, mix-fried Radix Glycyrrhizae (*Zhi Gan Cao*), 3g

2. Kidney heat & stomach dryness

Symptoms: Blackening of the teeth with grime, dry throat and mouth, vexation and agitation, insomnia, possible fullness in the abdomen and constipation, a crimson tongue, and a rapid pulse

Therapeutic principles: Clear the stomach and rescue the kidneys

Acupuncture & moxibustion:

Fu Liu (Ki 7) *San Yin Jiao* (Sp 6)	Together, these points nourish the stomach and also clear heat in the kidneys.
Xuan Zhong (GB 39) *Xia Ju Xu* (St 39)	Together, these points clear the stomach, while *Xuan Zhong* also replenishes the essence and engenders marrow.
Xue Hai (Sp 10)	Engenders the blood to moisten dryness and help engender essence

Additions & subtractions: If there is kidney essence depletion with loose teeth, pain and weakness of the low back and knees, hair loss, a dull, pale tongue with thin, white fur, and a deep, weak pulse, add *Tai Xi* (Ki 3), and *Shen Shu* (Bl 23).

Chinese medicinal formula: Modified *Yu Nu Jian* (Jade Maiden Decoction)

Ingredients: Uncooked Gypsum Fibrosum (*Shi Gao*), 18g, prepared Radix Rehmanniae (*Shu Di*), 18g, salt mix-fried Rhizoma Anemarrhenae Asphodeloidis (*Zhi Mu*), 9g, salt mix-fried Cortex Phellodendri (*Huang Bai*), 9g, salt stir-fried Radix Achyranthis Bidentatae (*Niu Xi*), 9g, Tuber Ophiopogonis Japonici (*Mai Men Dong*), 9g, Radix Scrophulariae Ningpoensis (*Xuan Shen*), 6g

Additions & subtractions: If there is kidney essence depletion with loose teeth, pain and weakness of the low back and knees, hair loss, a dull, pale tongue with thin, white fur, and a deep, weak pulse, add salt stir-fried Cortex Eucommiae Ulmoidis (*Du Zhong*), 9g, Rhizoma Drynariae (*Gu Sui Bu*), 9g, and Fructus Lycii Chinensis (*Gou Qi*), 9g, and increase the dosage of prepared Radix Rehmanniae (*Shu Di*).

35
Bruxism (*Yao Ya Nie Chi*)

Bruxism refers to unconsciously gritting or grinding the teeth, especially in stressful situations or during sleep.

Disease causes, disease mechanisms:

I. Exuberant fire of the heart & stomach

Heart fire may be due to excesses of the five affects, while the stomach fire may arise from addiction to alcohol and chilled, fatty, and/or rich-flavored food. If stomach fire stirs heart fire and these two flame upward in combination along the stomach channel that circles the mouth and enters the teeth, fire may stay in the network vessels there, leading to disquietude of the teeth. This is because fire is a yang evil and the nature of yang is to move. To comfort the teeth, there will be bruxism.

2. Accumulation & stagnation of food & drink

Dietary irregularities can damage the spleen leading to milk and food stagnation and indigestion. In that case, the stomach will become disharmonious. As it is said, "No harmony of the stomach, no sound sleep." With stomach disharmony, the teeth will become disquieted, since the stomach channel enters the teeth. Therefore, there may be bruxism during sleep.

3. Roundworms harassing internally

Unclean food intake may give rise to the engenderment of roundworms. If roundworms accumulate and harass internally, the stomach duct qi will fail to descend properly, thus leading to disharmony of the stomach qi. If there is stomach qi disharmony, the teeth will become disquieted, since the stomach channel enters the teeth. Therefore, there may be bruxism during sleep.

4. Qi & blood vacuity

Qi and blood vacuity can be due to constitutional spleen-stomach vacuity, enduring disease, and/or taxation. The normal movement of the jaws depends on healthy sinews of the jaw that are nourished and warmed by qi and blood. If there is qi and blood vacuity, the sinews cannot get sufficient nourishment and warming, and this may lead to inhibited movement of the jaws and then to bruxism.

5. Liver wind stirring internally

Wind may be due to liver-kidney yin vacuity from aging, enduring disease, late stage warm disease, excesses of the five affects, and sexual taxation where yin fails to check yang properly. The sinews depend on the liver, while the bones (and teeth) depend on the kidneys. In addition, wind is mobile by nature. Hence, if liver wind stirs internally, there may be bruxism during sleep.

Treatment based on pattern discrimination:

I. Exuberant fire of the heart & stomach

Symptoms: Grinding of the teeth with sound, vexation, bad breath, thirst with a liking for chilled drinks, swift digestion with rapid hungering, vomiting, clamoring stomach, possible immediate vomiting of undigested food, a red tongue with yellow fur lacking moisture, and a slippery, rapid pulse

Therapeutic principles: Clear the stomach and drain fire

Acupuncture & moxibustion:

Da Ling (Per 7)	Together, these points clear the heart and quiet the
Shen Men (Ht 7)	spirit. *Nei Guan* also helps *Zhong Wan* harmonize
Nei Guan (Per 6)	the stomach.

Zhong Wan (CV 12)	Together, these points drain fire and harmonize
Nei Ting (St 44)	the stomach.

Chinese medicinal formula: Modified *Qing Wei San* (Clear Stomach Powder)

Ingredients: Uncooked Gypsum Fibrosum (*Shi Gao*), 18g, wine stir-fried Rhizoma Coptidis Chinensis (*Huang Lian*), 6g, uncooked Radix Rehmanniae (*Sheng Di*), 15g, uncooked Radix Angelicae Sinensis (*Dang Gui*), 9g, Cortex Radicis Moutan (*Dan Pi*), 9g, uncooked Rhizoma Cimicifugae (*Sheng Ma*), 3g, Radix Glycyrrhizae (*Gan Cao*), 3g, Fructus Gardeniae Jasminoidis (*Zhi Zi*), 9g, Plumula Nelumbinis Nuciferae (*Lian Xin*), 3g

2. Accumulation & stagnation of food & drink

Symptoms: Grinding of the teeth during sleep, insomnia, glomus and oppression in the chest and stomach, no thought for food, indigestion, fatigued spirit, inhibited defecation, diarrhea with abdominal pain, or constipation, dark-colored urine, slimy and slightly yellow tongue fur, and a slippery, replete pulse

Therapeutic principles: Disperse food, abduct stagnation, and harmonize the center

Acupuncture and moxibustion:

Jiu Wei (CV 15)	Harmonizes the stomach and quiets the heart
Xia Wan (CV 10)	Downbears the stomach qi to harmonize the stomach
Xuan Ji (CV 21)	An empirical point for dispersing food
Zu San Li (St 36)	Fortifies the spleen to transform the food

Additions & subtractions: For cold pain in the abdomen, add *Shen Que* (CV 8) with moxibustion.

Chinese medicinal formula: Modified *Bao He Wan* (Preserve Harmony Pills)

Ingredients: Stir-fried Fructus Crataegi (*Shan Zha*), 9g, stir-fried Fructus Germinatus Hordei Vulgaris (*Mai Ya*), 9g, stir-fried Massa Medica Fermentata (*Shen Qu*), 9g, stir-fried Pericarpium Citri Reticulatae (*Chen Pi*), 9g, Sclerotium Poriae Cocos (*Fu Ling*), 9g, Fructus Forsythiae Suspensae (*Lian Qiao*), 9g, Semen Raphani Sativi (*Lai Fu Zi*), 9g, Fructus Citri Aurantii (*Zhi Ke*), 6g, lime-processed Rhizoma Pinelliae Ternatae (*Ban Xia*), 9g, Semen Panici Miliacei (*Shu Mi*), 9g

3. Roundworms harassing internally

Symptoms: Grinding of the teeth during sleep, glomus in the stomach, intermittent abdominal pain, dirty habits, such as not washing one's hands before eating, addictions to peculiar foods, a sallow facial complexion, emaciation, possible itching in the nostrils, blue macules or speckles in the whites of the eyes, roundworm macules of white color on the face, translucent milliary eruptions on the inside of the lips, bright red speckled eruptions on the tip of the tongue or on the sides of the midline of the tongue, a pale red tongue with white fur, and a wiry, slippery pulse

Therapeutic principles: Expel the roundworms, fortify the spleen, and transform dampness

Acupuncture & moxibustion:

Zhong Wan (CV 12) *Da Heng* (Sp 15)	Together, these points move the spleen, harmonize the stomach, and free the qi mechanism.
Nei Guan (Per 6) *Gong Sun* (Sp 4)	Together, these points loosen the center, downbear the qi, and quiet the roundworms.
Zu San Li (St 36)	Fortifies the spleen and transforms dampness
Bai Chong Wo (M-LE-34)	An empirical point for expelling roundworms

Chinese medicinal formula: *Wu Mei Wan* (Mume Pills)

Ingredients: Uncooked Fructus Pruni Mume (*Wu Mei*), 9g, Radix Codonopsitis Pilosulae (*Dang Shen*), 6g, Herba Asari Cum Radice (*Xi Xin*), 3g, uncooked Cortex Phellodendri (*Huang Bai*), 6g, processed Radix Lateralis Praeparatus Aconiti Carmichaeli (*Fu Zi*), 3g, stir-fried Ramulus Cinnamomi Cassiae (*Gui Zhi*), 3g, uncooked Rhizoma Coptidis Chinensis (*Huang Lian*), 6g, dry Rhizoma Zingiberis (*Gan Jiang*), 6g, uncooked Radix Angelicae Sinensis (*Dang Gui*), 6g, Pericarpium Zanthoxyli Bungeani (*Chuan Jiao*), 3g

4. Qi & blood vacuity

Symptoms: Grinding of the teeth with low sound, a bright pale facial complexion, reduced qi with disinclination to speak, pale lips and nails, dizziness and vertigo, heart palpitations, tinnitus, a fat, pale tongue with thin, white fur, and a fine, weak or vacuous, large pulse

Therapeutic principles: Boost the qi and nourish the blood

Acupuncture & moxibustion:

Zu San Li (St 36) *San Yin Jiao* (Sp 6)	Together, these points fortify the spleen to enhance the source of engendering and transforming the qi and blood.
Xin Shu (Bl 15) *Pi Shu* (Bl 20) *Ge Shu* (Bl 17)	Together, these points nourish the blood.

Chinese medicinal formula: Modified *Ba Zhen Tang* (Eight Pearls Decoction)

Ingredients: Prepared Radix Rehmanniae (*Shu Di*), 12g, Radix Angelicae Sinensis (*Dang Gui*), 9g, Radix Albus Paeoniae Lactiflorae (*Bai Shao*), 15g, uncooked Radix Ligustici Wallichii (*Chuan Xiong*), 6g, honey stir-fried Radix Codonopsitis Pilosulae (*Dang Shen*), 9g, bran stir-fried Rhizoma Atractylodis Macrocephalae (*Bai Zhu*), 9g, Sclerotium Poriae Cocos (*Fu Ling*), 9g, mix-fried Radix Glycyrrhizae (*Zhi Gan Cao*), 6g, Caulis Milletiae Seu Spatholobi (*Ji Xue Teng*), 12g

5. Liver wind stirring internally

Symptoms: Grinding of the teeth with sound, tremors of the hands and feet, convulsions in severe case, redness above the cheekbones, night sweats, vexatious heat in the five hearts, dry mouth and throat, a red tongue with little moisture, and a fine, rapid, deep pulse

Therapeutic principles: Nourish liver-kidney yin and subdue yang, extinguish wind and stop tremors

Acupuncture & moxibustion:

Tai Chong (Liv 3) *Feng Chi* (GB 20)	Together, these points subdue yang, extinguish the wind, and stop tremors.

Tai Xi (Ki 3)   Together, these points nourish yin.
San Yin Jiao (Sp 6)

Chinese medicinal formula: *Zhen Gan Xi Feng Tang* (Settle the Liver & Extinguish Wind Decoction)

Ingredients: Uncooked Haemititum (*Dai Zhe Shi*), 18g, salt stir-fried Radix Achyranthis Bidentatae (*Niu Xi*), 18g, uncooked Os Draconis (*Long Gu*), 15g, uncooked Concha Ostreae (*Mu Li*), 15g, uncooked Plastrum Testudinis (*Gui Ban*), 15g, Radix Scrophulariae Ningpoensis (*Xuan Shen*), 9g, Tuber Asparagi Cochinensis (*Tian Men Dong*), 9g, uncooked Radix Albus Paeoniae Lactiflorae (*Bai Shao*), 15g, Herba Artemisiae Capillaris (*Yin Chen Hao*), 6g, Fructus Meliae Toosendan (*Chuan Lian Zi*), 6g, Fructus Germinatus Hordei Vulgaris (*Mai Ya*), 6g, Radix Glycyrrhizae (*Gan Cao*), 6g

Note: Bruxism is a common symptom amongst Western female patients who may either say they have "TMJ" or that they grind their teeth at night. They may also say that their dentist has fitted them with a mouth splint to wear at night during sleep. Commonly, such women also suffer from neck and shoulder tension and restless sleep or insomnia, possibly with profuse dreams. Typically, such women in their late 30s and throughout their 40s present a more complex pattern than the simple patterns described above. Frequently, they display a combination of spleen vacuity leading to qi and blood vacuity, liver depression with depressive heat, and an element of underlying kidney vacuity. Usually they do not manifest full-blown signs and symptoms of liver wind.

36
Tooth Pain (*Ya Tong*)

This refers to pain of the teeth. It is often accompanied by painful, swollen gums.

Disease causes, disease mechanisms:

I. Wind heat

Wind heat is mainly due to contraction of external wind heat. Heat is a yang evil which flames upward by nature. If wind and heat flame upward together, congesting in the network vessels that connect with the teeth, there will be inhibited flow of qi and blood in addition to the burning of the heat. "Lack of free flow leads to pain" and, therefore, there is pain in the teeth.

2. Wind cold

Wind cold is mostly due to external contraction. When wind attacks, due to its inherently yang nature, it tends to affect the upper body first. Cold evils are congealing by nature and are associated with contraction. If wind and cold invade the body together and congest in the network vessels that connect with the teeth, there will be contraction followed by inhibited flow of the qi and blood, thus leading to tooth pain.

3. Stomach fire

Stomach heat is mainly due to a hot constitution coupled with addiction to spicy, acrid, dry food or alcohol that engender heat. If heat accumulates in the stomach, it will fume and then steam upward along the stomach channel to the teeth. Heat steaming and congesting in the network vessels of the teeth will then lead to pain of the teeth.

4. Vacuity fire

Vacuity fire may arise from aging or unrestrained sexual activity leading to kidney yin vacuity. Being vacuous, kidney yin cannot check yang properly, thus giving rise to yin vacuity fire. If this fire flares upward, it will burn the network vessels that connect with the teeth, resulting in tooth pain.

5. Qi vacuity

Qi vacuity may be the result of taxation or enduring diseases that consume the qi. Qi is responsible for moving the blood. As it is said, "If the qi moves, the blood moves." If the qi becomes vacuous, it may fail to push the blood and move it upward to fill the network vessels that connect with the teeth. This will then lead to disharmony and undernourishment of these vessels. Since the qi and blood do not move freely in the local area, there is pain in the teeth.

6. Tooth decay

Tooth decay can be from addiction to fatty meat, fine grain, and strong flavours or sweet food whose residue may be left in between the teeth and engender a swarm of "teeth worms", (*i.e.*, germs). When these teeth worms chew on and damage the teeth, there will be toothache.

Treatment based on pattern discrimination:

I. Wind heat

Symptoms: Distention and pain in the teeth which is worsened by heat or spicy food and is ameliorated by cold, distended, swollen gums, inability to chew food, possibly a hot, swollen cheek, thirst, a red tongue tip with thin, white or slightly yellow, dry fur, and a floating, rapid pulse

Therapeutic principles: Course wind, clear heat, and stop pain

Acupuncture & moxibustion:

Wai Guan (TB 5) *Feng Chi* (GB 20)	Together, these points course wind and resolve the exterior.
He Gu (LI 4) *Xia Guan* (St 7) *Jia Che* (St 6)	Together, these points clear heat in the *yang ming* to stop pain.
Jiao Sun (TB 20)	An intersection point of the triple burner, gall-bladder, and large intestine channels which clears heat and stops pain. Direct the tip of the needle toward *Tai Yang* (M-HN-9).

Note: Use the points on the affected side only.

Additions & subtractions: For headache in the temples, add *Tai Yang* (M-HN-9). For fever, add *Da Zhui* (GV 14). For pain in front of the ear, add *Er Men* (TB 21) or *Ting Hui* (GB 2). For pain behind the ear, add *Yi Feng* (TB 17). For pain in the lower teeth, add *Da Ying* (St 5). For pain in the upper teeth, add *Jiao Sun* (TB 20). Other points may be similarly added depending on the location and accompanying signs and symptoms.

Chinese medicinal formula: Modified *Huang Lian Shang Qing Wan* (Coptis Upper [Burner] Clearing Pills)

Ingredients: Radix Ledebouriellae Divaricatae (*Fang Feng*), 6g, Herba Menthae Haplocalysis (*Bo He*), 3g, Herba Schizonepetae Tenuifoliae (*Jing Jie*), 6g, Radix Angelicae Dahuricae (*Bai Zhi*), 6g, wine stir-fried Rhizoma Coptidis Chinensis (*Huang Lian*), 3g, uncooked Cortex Phellodendri (*Huang Bai*), 3g, wine stir-fried Radix Scutellariae Baicalensis (*Huang Qin*), 3g, Fructus Gardeniae Jasminoidis (*Zhi Zi*), 3g, uncooked Gypsum Fibrosum (*Shi Gao*), 20g, Fructus Forsythiae

Suspensae (*Lian Qiao*), 6g, Radix Et Rhizoma Rhei (*Da Huang*), 3g, Herba Asari Cum Radice (*Xi Xin*), 3g

Additions & subtractions: If there is oppression of the chest, add Herba Agastachis Seu Pogostemi (*Huo Xiang*), 9g, and Tuber Curcumae (*Yu Jin*), 9g. If there is swollen, painful throat, add Fructus Aristolochiae (*Ma Dou Ling*), 9g, Fructus Arctii Lappae (*Niu Bang Zi*), 12g, and Radix Scrophulariae Ningpoensis (*Xuan Shen*), 9g. If the gums are bleeding, subtract Herba Schizonepetae Tenuifoliae (*Jing Jie*) and add Rhizoma Imperatae Cylindricae (*Bai Mao Gen*), 9g, Cacumen Biotae Orientalis (*Ce Bai Ye*), 9g, and Fructus Gardeniae Jasminoidis (*Zhi Zi*), 9g.

2. Wind cold

Symptoms: Paroxysmal pain in the teeth worsened by inhalation of cold air and ameliorated by heat, aversion to wind and cold, no thirst, a pale red tongue with thin, white fur, and a floating, tight, or slow pulse

Therapeutic principles: Course wind, dissipate cold, and stop pain

Acupuncture & moxibustion:

Shang Yang (LI 1) *He Gu* (LI 4)	Together, these points course wind and dissipate cold.
Xia Guan (St 7) *Jia Che* (St 6)	Together, these points course and unblock the network vessels to stop the pain.

Additions & subtractions: For aversion to cold, add *Wai Guan* (TB 5). See the additions & subtractions for the wind heat pattern above and follow the same methodology.

Chinese medicinal formula: Modified *Ma Huang Fu Zi Xi Xin Tang* (Ephedra, Aconite & Asarum Decoction)

Ingredients: Uncooked Herba Ephedrae (*Ma Huang*), 6g, bland Radix Lateralis Praeparatus Aconiti Carmichaeli (*Fu Zi*), 3g, Herba Asari Cum Radice (*Xi Xin*), 3g, Radix Angelicae Dahuricae (*Bai Zhi*), 9g, Radix Et Rhizoma Ligustici Chinensis (*Gao Ben*), 9g

Additions & subtractions: If toothache is severe, add Radix Puerariae (*Ge Gen*), 9g, Radix Ligustici Wallichii (*Chuan Xiong*), 9g, and Fructus Piperis Longi (*Bi Ba*), 3g.

3. Stomach fire

Symptoms: Distention and pain in the teeth which may involve the head, possible red, swollen gums, hot face, thirst with a desire for chilled drinks, hot, bad breath, a liking for cold with a dislike for heat, possible painful, swollen lips, tongue, and cheeks, constipation, dark-colored urine, a red, dry tongue with yellow fur, and a surging, rapid or slippery, rapid pulse

Therapeutic principles: Clear and drain heat, stop pain

Acupuncture & moxibustion:

He Gu (LI 4) *Nei Ting* (St 44)	Together, these points clear and drain heat in the *yang ming*.
Xia Guan (St 7) *Tai Yang* (M-HN-9) *Tou Wei* (St 8)	Together, these points course and free the network vessels to stop pain.
Feng Long (St 40)	Frees the stools and drains heat

Additions & subtractions: For frontal headache, add *Yin Tang* (M-HN-3). For pain in the lower teeth, add *Da Ying* (St 5). For pain in the upper teeth, add *Jiao Sun* (TB 20).

Chinese medicinal formula: Modified *Qing Wei San* (Clear the Stomach Powder)

Ingredients: Uncooked Gypsum Fibrosum (*Shi Gao*), 24g, wine stir-fried Rhizoma Coptidis Chinensis (*Huang Lian*), 6g, uncooked Radix Rehmanniae (*Sheng Di*), 9g, uncooked Radix Angelicae Sinensis (*Dang Gui*), 9g, Cortex Radicis Moutan (*Dan Pi*), 9g, uncooked Rhizoma Cimicifugae (*Sheng Ma*), 6g, Radix Glycyrrhizae (*Gan Cao*), 3g, Rhizoma Anemarrhenae Asphodeloidis (*Zhi Mu*), 9g, Radix Cyathulae (*Chuan Niu Xi*), 9g, Radix Scrophulariae Ningpoensis (*Xuan Shen*), 9g, Radix Angelicae Dahuricae (*Bai Zhi*), 9g

Additions & subtractions: If toothache is severe, add Herba Asari Cum Radice (*Xi Xin*), 3g, and Radix Seu Rhizoma Cynanchi (*Xu Chang Qing*), 9g. If there is concomitant kidney yin vacuity, subtract uncooked Radix Rehmanniae (*Sheng Di*) and Radix Cyathulae (*Chuan Niu Xi*) and add prepared Radix Rehmanniae (*Shu Di*), 18g, Radix Achyranthis Bidentatae (*Niu Xi*), 9g, and Tuber Ophiopogonis Japonici (*Mai Men Dong*), 9g.

4. Vacuity fire

Symptoms: Dull pain in the teeth, loose teeth, red lips and cheeks, dry, sore throat, heart palpitations, dizziness, vacuity vexation, insomnia, pain and weakness of the low back and spine, a red tongue with reduced fluids and fur, and a fine, rapid pulse

Therapeutic principles: Enrich yin, supplement the kidneys, and stop pain

Acupuncture & moxibustion:

Tai Xi (Ki 3)	Together, these points enrich yin and supplement
Fu Liu (Ki 7)	the kidneys.
Quan Liao (SI 18)	Courses and frees the network vessels to stop pain
Tong Li (Ht 5)	Clears sovereign fire

Additions & subtractions: For headache at the vertex, add *Bai Hui* (GV 20). For pain in the lower teeth, add *Da Ying* (St 5). For pain in the upper teeth, add *Jiao Sun* (TB 20).

Chinese medicinal formula: Modified *Zhi Bai Di Huang Wan* (Anemarrhena & Phellodendron Rehmannia Pills)

Ingredients: Prepared Radix Rehmanniae (*Shu Di*), 18g, steamed Fructus Corni Officinalis (*Shan Zhu Yu*), 9g, Sclerotium Poriae Cocos (*Fu Ling*), 6g, salt mix-fried Rhizoma Alismatis (*Ze Xie*), 6g, Cortex Radicis Moutan (*Dan Pi*), 12g, salt mix-fried Rhizoma Anemarrhenae Asphodeloidis (*Zhi Mu*), 9g, salt mix-fried Cortex Phellodendri (*Huang Bai*), 9g, Cortex Radicis Lycii Chinensis (*Di Gu Pi*), 9g, salt stir-fried Radix Achyranthis Bidentatae (*Niu Xi*), 9g, Rhizoma Drynariae (*Gu Sui Bu*), 9g, Cortex Cinnamomi Cassiae (*Rou Gui*), 1g

5. Qi vacuity

Symptoms: Lingering, dull pain in the teeth, a pale, fat tongue with thin, white, or white fur, slightly red, swollen gums or gums which are swollen but not red, a bright pale facial complexion, reduced qi with disinclination to speak, speaking in a low voice, fatigue and lack of strength, spontaneous sweating, heart palpitations, dizziness, tinnitus, frequent, clear urination weak or vacuous, large pulse

Therapeutic principles: Supplement the qi and stop pain

Acupuncture & moxibustion:

He Gu (LI 4)	Together, these points supplement the qi and stop
Zu San Li (St 36)	pain when moxa is burned on the handles of the needles.

Additions & subtractions: For speaking in a low voice, add *Shan Zhong* (CV 17).

Chinese medicinal formula: Modified *Bu Zhong Yi Qi Tang* (Supplement the Center & Boost the Qi Decoction)

Ingredients: Honey stir-fried Radix Astragali Membranacei (*Huang Qi*), 15g, mix-fried Radix Glycyrrhizae (*Zhi Gan Cao*), 6g, honey stir-fried Radix Codonopsitis Pilosulae (*Dang Shen*), 9g, bran stir-fried Rhizoma Atractylodis Macrocephalae (*Bai Zhu*), 6g, stir-fried Radix Angelicae Sinensis (*Dang Gui*), 9g, stir-fried Pericarpium Citri Reticulatae (*Chen Pi*), 6g, honey mix-fried Rhizoma Cimicifugae (*Sheng Ma*), 3g, stir-fried Radix Bupleuri (*Chai Hu*), 3g, Sclerotium Poriae Cocos (*Fu Ling*), 12g, Herba Asari Cum Radice (*Xi Xin*), 3g, Fructus Piperis Longi (*Bi Ba*), 3g, Radix Angelicae Dahuricae (*Bai Zhi*), 9g, Radix Seu Rhizoma Cynanchi (*Xu Chang Qing*), 9g

6. Tooth decay

Symptoms: Intermittent toothache, severe pain when there is a stimulant like pressure or when cold or warm drinks touch the site of decay, and no other obvious symptoms

Therapeutic principles: Clear heat and stop pain

Acupuncture & moxibustion:

He Gu (LI 4)	Courses and unblocks the channel qi to stop the pain
Chong Yang (St 42) *Tai Chong* (Liv 3)	Together, these points clear heat.

Note: For the above pattern of toothache, acupuncture can only relieve the pain for a little while or it may be completely ineffective. Therefore, a combined therapy is suggested.

Chinese medicinal formula: The following unnamed formula is effective for pain but does not treat the real cause of the disease.

Ingredients: Fructus Piperis Longi (*Bi Ba*), 20g, Pericarpium Zanthoxyli Bungeani (*Chuan Jiao*), 20g, Herba Asari Cum Radice (*Xi Xin*), 20g, Flos Caryophylli (*Ding Xiang*), 20g.

Put the powdered medicinals in the affected area.

Remarks: Many Chinese medicinals achieve a good effect for toothache. However, it is important to know their differences and how to prescribe them. For instance, Herba Asari Cum Radice (*Xi Xin*) is a powerful analgesic for tooth pain, but it is mainly effective for wind conditions (wind heat and wind cold) and is mainly used externally in powder form. Radix Angelicae Dahuricae (*Bai Zhu*) is also an effective Chinese medicinal for wind conditions and especially for wind cold with tooth pain and swollen gums. It is both applied externally and administered orally. Traditionally, Angelica Dahurica is often used to treat the upper teeth, while Asarum is often used to treat the lower teeth. Nevertheless, in all cases, Asarum is stronger for treating toothache even for the upper teeth. However, in such cases, it is only applied externally in powdered form.

Radix Angelicae Pubescentis (*Du Huo*) is effective when headache refers to the teeth. Rhizoma Drynariae (*Gu Sui Bu*) is the best Chinese medicinal when the condition is a kidney vacuity. It is used internally. Cortex Radicis Lycii Chinensis (*Di Gu Pi*) is effective when vacuity fire from kidney vacuity conterflows upwards. It is used internally.
Rhizoma Cimicifugae (*Sheng Ma*) is the typical Chinese medicinal prescribed when there is fire depression. It is the indispensable messenger medicinal in a classic formula that clears heat and drains fire in the stomach. It is used internally.

Radix Et Rhizoma Rhei (*Da Huang*) is also a key medicinal for toothache due to replete heat in the *yang ming* accompanied by constipation. It strongly increases therapeutic results and is used internally. Gypsum Fibrosum (*Shi Gao*) is a classic Chinese medicinal for stomach fire and is used internally.

Herba Pycnostelmae (*Xu Chang Jing*) is a relatively little known Chinese medicinal. It is a powerful analgesic for many disorders where pain is the main complaint, as in toothache. For this problem, it is especially used, both internally and externally, for wind conditions.

37

Pain & Swelling of the Gums (*Ya Yin Zhong Tong*)

This refers to topical redness, pain, and swelling of the affected gum. In its early stage, the topical area is hard and then becomes soft. The patient feels that the tooth located in the affected area is longer than usual and it hurts when touched. In the late stage, the teeth become loose and there are fissures in the gum which drain pus. The cheek can also be involved, manifested by distention and swelling.

Disease causes, disease mechanisms:

I. Wind heat external invasion

When external wind heat invades the body, it may stir accumulated spleen-stomach heat. If this combined heat steams and flames upward to the gums along the channel, it will burn and damage the network vessels in the gums, resulting in painful, swollen gums.

2. Foul toxin binding & depression

Addiction to sweet and/or sour food or poor dental hygiene may lead to tooth decay. Foul toxins may thus be engendered which accumulate in the gums or around the roots of the teeth. There they putrefy the flesh, leading to painful swelling of the gums followed by suppuration.

3. Exuberant spleen-stomach fire

Exuberant spleen-stomach fire may arise from addiction to alcohol and/or spicy food that engenders heat. Accumulating and brewing in the center, this heat may transform into fire. If this fire flames upward to the gums, it will burn, damage, and putrefy the flesh and network vessels of the gums, leading to painful swelling of the gums.

4. Qi & blood vacuity

Enduring pain and swelling of the gums with suppuration may consume the qi and blood and cause qi and blood vacuity. In such cases, the opening of the affected area is difficult to heal since the vacuous qi and blood fail to dispel the evils. Therefore, the pain and swelling of the gums may develop into gum fistula.

Treatment based on pattern discrimination:

I. Wind heat external invasion

Symptoms: Red, hard, painful, swollen gums with burning heat, aversion to cold, fever, headache, a red tongue with thin, yellow fur, and a floating, rapid pulse

Therapeutic principles: Course wind and clear heat, resolve toxins and disperse swelling

Acupuncture & moxibustion:

Jiao Sun (TB 20) *Hai* (SI 8)	This is a classic formula for painful gums. *Xiao* Together, these points clear heat, disperse swelling, and stop pain.
He Gu (LI 4) *Wen Liu* (LI 7)	Together, these points course wind, clear heat, and resolve toxins.

Additions & subtractions: For fever, add *Da Zhui* (GV 14). For frontal headache, add *Tou Wei* (St 8). For occipital headache, add *Feng Chi* (GB 20).

Chinese medicinal formula: Modified *Wu Wei Xiao Du Yin* (Five Flavors Disperse Toxins Drink)

Ingredients: Flos Lonicerae Japonicae (*Jin Yin Hua*), 15g, Flos Chrysanthemi Indici (*Ye Ju Hua*), 12g, Herba Taraxaci Mongolici Cum Radice (*Pu Gong Ying*), 9g, Herba Violae Yedoensitis Cum Radice (*Zi Hua Di Ding*), 9g, Radix Semiaquilegiae (*Tian Kui Zi*), 9g, Radix Ledebouriellae Divaricatae (*Fang Feng*), 9g, Fructus Forsythiae Suspensae (*Lian Qiao*), 9g, Herba Menthae Haplocalysis (*Bo He*), 3g, Radix Scutellariae Baicalensis (*Huang Qin*), 6g

2. Foul toxin binding & depression

Symptoms: Red, hard, swollen gums following enduring tooth decay, abscess in the gums followed by discharge of pus

Therapeutic principles: Clear heat and resolve toxins

Acupuncture & moxibustion:

Cheng Jiang (CV 24)	Clears heat in the local area and stops pain
Lao Gong (Per 8) *He Gu* (LI 4)	Together, these points unblock the channels and drain heat.
Guan Chong (TB 1) *Zhong Chong* (Per 9)	Together, these points clear heat and resolve toxins when pricked to bleed.

Chinese medicinal formula: Modified *Wu Wei Xiao Du Yin* (Five Flavors Disperse Toxins Drink)

Ingredients: Flos Lonicerae Japonicae (*Jin Yin Hua*), 15g, Flos Chrysanthemi Indici (*Ye Ju Hua*), 12g, Herba Taraxaci Mongolici Cum Radice (*Pu Gong Ying*), 9g, Herba Violae Yedoensitis Cum Radice (*Zi Hua Di Ding*), 9g, Radix Semiaquilegiae (*Tian Kui Zi*), 9g, Fructus Forsythiae Suspensae (*Lian Qiao*), 9g, wine stir-fried Radix Scutellariae Baicalensis (*Huang Qin*), 6g, wine stir-fried Rhizoma Coptidis Chinensis (*Huang Lian*), 6g, Fructus Gardeniae Jasminoidis (*Zhi Zi*), 9g

3. Exuberant spleen-stomach fire

Symptoms: Topical pain and distention of the gum extending to the cheek, a bitter taste in the mouth, bad breath, a red tongue with yellow fur, and a rapid pulse

Therapeutic principles: Clear the stomach and drain fire

Acupuncture & moxibustion:

Jia Che (St 6)	Clears heat in the local area and unblocks the network vessels
He Gu (LI 4) *Qu Chi* (LI 11)	Together, these points clear large intestine heat.
Nei Ting (St 44) *Da Du* (Sp 2)	Together, these points clear the stomach and drain fire.

Additions & subtractions: For persistent bad breath, add *Da Ling* (Per 7) or *Lao Gong* (Per 8). For constipation, add *Shang Ju Xu* (St 37) and *Tian Shu* (St 25). For a bitter taste in the mouth, add *Yang Ling Quan* (GB 34).

Chinese medicinal formula: Modified *Qing Wei Tang* (Clear the Stomach Decoction)

Ingredients: Uncooked Gypsum Fibrosum (*Shi Gao*), 24g, wine stir-fried Radix Scutellariae Baicalensis (*Huang Qin*), 9g, wine stir-fried Rhizoma Coptidis Chinensis (*Huang Lian*), 6g, uncooked Radix Rehmanniae (*Sheng Di*), 12g, Cortex Radicis Moutan (*Dan Pi*), 9g, uncooked Rhizoma Cimicifugae (*Sheng Ma*), 6g, Radix Glycyrrhizae (*Gan Cao*), 3g

4. Qi & blood vacuity

Symptoms: Painful swelling of the gum with fissuring which occasionally discharges pus. The opening is difficult to heal. In addition, there is a pale tongue and a fine, weak pulse.

Therapeutic principles: Draw out the toxins and engender the muscles (*i.e.*, flesh)

Acupuncture & moxibustion:

He Gu (LI 4)	Together, these points supplement the qi to draw
Zu San Li (St 36)	out the toxins and engender the muscles (*i.e.*, flesh).
San Yin Jiao (Sp 6)	Together, these points fortify the spleen to
Xue Hai (Sp 10)	engender the blood.

Chinese medicinal formula: Modified *Tuo Li Xiao Du San* (Support the Interior & Disperse Toxins Powder)

Ingredients: Honey stir-fried Radix Codonopsitis Pilosulae (*Dang Shen*), 9g, bran stir-fried Rhizoma Atractylodis Macrocephalae (*Bai Zhu*), 9g, uncooked Radix Astragali Membranacei (*Huang Qi*), 15g, wine mix-fried Radix Ligustici Wallichii (*Chuan Xiong*), 9g, wine mix-fried Radix Angelicae Sinensis (*Dang Gui*), 9g, Squama Manitis Pentadactylis (*Chuan Shan Jia*), 6g, Radix Angelicae Dahuricae (*Bai Zhi*), 6g, Rhizoma Cimicifugae (*Sheng Ma*), 3g, Spina Gleditschiae Chinensis (*Zao Jiao Ci*), 9g, mix-fried Radix Glycyrrhizae (*Zhi Gan Cao*), 6g

38
Putrefying Gums (*Ya Yin Fu Lan*)

Putrefying gums are also known as *gan* of the teeth. This refers to putrefied flesh and blood in the affected gum(s) which may slough off , bleed, and/or discharge pus.

Disease causes, disease mechanisms:

I. Wind heat

Wind and heat in this condition are external evils. "Wind is a yang evil that tends to attack the upper body", while "Heat is a yang evil that tends to flame upward." When wind heat strikes a body where there is already stomach heat accumulation, this wind and heat may stir up the accumulated heat which then together attacks the gums, remembering that the stomach channel enters the teeth. If wind and heat together with accumulated stomach heat congest in the gums, they will burn and then putrefy the flesh and qi and blood in the gums, leading to putrefying gums.

2. Epidemic toxins

In late stage febrile disease, the correct qi is often vacuous. If seasonal epidemic toxins take advantage of this vacuity to invade the body, they may congest in the gums and putrefy the flesh and qi and blood in the gums, resulting in *gan* of the teeth.

3. Exuberant internal heat

Exuberant internal heat may be due to excesses of the five affects or addiction to alcohol or spicy, fatty, rich food. Once exuberant, first this heat may cause frenetic movement of the blood, thus leading to bleeding. Secondly, it may transform into fire toxins, resulting in putrefying of the gums if these fire toxins congest therein.

Treatment based on pattern discrimination:

I. Wind heat *gan* of the teeth & gums

Symptoms: Red, painful, swollen gums in the first 2-3 days, followed by erosion of the gums covered by a greyish white pseudo-membrane that is easy to scrape off, bad breath, increased saliva that is thick and sticky, poor appetite, intermittent fever and chills, nausea and vomiting, constipation, possible fever, headache, fatigued spirit, dark-colored urine, constipation when the erosion involves the soft palate, the root of the tongue, and the cheeks, possible painful, distended nodules in the neck that can be worse on pressure, yellow tongue fur, and a slippery, rapid pulse

Therapeutic principles: Course wind, clear heat, and resolve toxins

Acupuncture & moxibustion:

Ren Zhong (GV 26)   Clears heat

Shang Yang (LI 1)   Together, these points course wind and clear heat.
He Gu (LI 4)
Wai Guan (TB 5)

Wei Zhong (Bl 40)   Clears heat and resolves toxins when pricked to
                        bleed

Additions & subtractions: For high fever, add *Qu Chi* (LI 11) and *Da Zhui* (GV 14). For intermittent fever and chills, add *Zhi Gou* (TB 6) and *Da Zhui* (GV 14).

Note: For *gan* of the teeth and gums, combined therapy is suggested, not just acupuncture alone.

Chinese medicinal formula: Modified *Qing Wei Tang* (Clear the Stomach Decoction)

Ingredients: Uncooked Gypsum Fibrosum (*Shi Gao*), 24g, wine stir-fried Radix Scutellariae Baicalensis (*Huang Qin*), 9g, wine stir-fried Rhizoma Coptidis Chinensis (*Huang Lian*), 6g, uncooked Radix Rehmanniae (*Sheng Di*), 12g, Cortex Radicis Moutan (*Dan Pi*), 9g, uncooked Rhizoma Cimicifugae (*Sheng Ma*), 6g, Radix Glycyrrhizae (*Gan Cao*), 3g, Herba Taraxaci Mongolici Cum Radice (*Pu Gong Ying*), 9g, Flos Chrysanthemi Indici (*Ye Ju Hua*), 9g

2. Galloping *gan* of the teeth & gums

Symptoms: This starts with a red, painful, swollen lump in the gum or in the cheek that becomes putrid in 1-2 days. At first, the putrid area is a greyish white color but soon turns black and hard. From this, a purple-black foul discharge drains. When the lesion softens, it sloughs off and the local site is itchy with slight pain. In 4-5 days, the erosion deepens, possibly involving the nose, the areas beside the nose, the cheeks and/or the lips. The site of erosion takes on a bluish brown color and may cause falling out of the teeth, perforation of the lips and cheeks, or collapse of the bridge of the nose. General symptoms may include high fever, clouded spirit, a red crimson tongue with yellow, slimy fur, and a fine, rapid pulse.

Symptoms such as panting, phlegm rales in the throat, and cold sweating from the forehead suggest deterioration, while symptoms like pink flesh instead of black sloughing at the site of erosion and bleeding a fresh blood suggest recovery.

Therapeutic principles: Clear heat and resolve toxins

Acupuncture & moxibustion:

Wei Zhong (Bl 40)	Together, these points clear heat and resolve
Shi Xuan (M-UE-1)	toxins when pricked to bleed.

Additions & subtractions: For high fever, add *Da Zhui* (GV 14). For clouded spirit, add *Ren Zhong* (GV 26). For cold sweating from the forehead, add *Shen Que* (CV 8) with moxibustion, *Zu San Li* (St 36), and *He Gu* (LI 4).

Note: For *gan* of the teeth and gums, acupuncture should be combined with internal medicine. Acupuncture alone is not recommended.

Chinese medicinal formula: Modified *Xi Jiao Di Huang Tang* (Rhinoceros Horn & Rehmannia Decoction)[10]

Ingredients: Cornu Bubali (*Shui Niu Jiao*), 20g, uncooked Radix Rehmanniae (*Sheng Di*), 30g, uncooked Radix Rubrus Paeoniae Lactiflorae (*Chi Shao*), 12g, Cortex Radicis Moutan (*Dan Pi*), 9g, uncooked Radix Scutellariae Baicalensis (*Huang Qin*), 9g, uncooked Rhizoma Coptidis Chinensis (*Huang Lian*), 6g, Fructus Gardeniae Jasminoidis (*Zhi Zi*), 9g, Herba Taraxaci Mongolici Cum Radice (*Pu Gong Ying*), 9g, Herba Violae Yedoensitis Cum Radice (*Zi Hua Di Ding*), 9g

---

[10] Blue Poppy Press does not advocate the use of medicinals manufactured from parts of endangered species. In this formula it is suitable to relace the Rhinoceros Horn with Water Buffalo Horn (Cornu Bubali, *Shuai Niu Jiao*)

3. Green-legged *gan* of the teeth & gums

Symptoms: Distended, swollen gums, erosion with discharge of pus and blood, perforation of the cheeks and lips in severe cases. This is accompanied by pain in the legs and lumps of different sizes which are greenish black in color, are hard, are located in the muscles of the legs. There may also be inhibited movement, body aches, and no sweating. There is puffy edema of the limbs and short voidings of clear urine when there is predominant cold dampness. There is also a bitter taste in the mouth, dry mouth, bad breath, a red tongue with yellow, dry fur, and a slippery, rapid pulse.

Therapeutic principles: Clear fire and resolve toxins

Acupuncture & moxibustion:

Wei Zhong (Bl 40) *Nu Xi* (M-LE-9)	Togther, these points clear fire and resolve toxins when pricked to bleed.
Yong Quan (Ki 1) *Nei Ting* (St 44)	Together, these points lead fire downward and drain fire.

Additions & subtractions: For puffy edema of the limbs and short voidings of clear urine, add *Zhong Ji* (CV 3) and *Yin Ling Quan* (Sp 9). For a bitter tastes in the mouth, add *Yang Ling Quan* (GB 34).

Note: As stated above, for *gan* of the teeth and gums, acupuncture should be combined with internal medicine.

Chinese medicinal formula: Modified *Huo Luo Liu Qi Yin* (Quicken the Network Vessels & Flow the Qi Drink)

Ingredients: Bran stir-fried Rhizoma Atractylodis (*Cang Zhu*), 9g, stir-fried Fructus Chaenomelis Lagenariae (*Mu Gua*), 9g, Radix Et Rhizoma Notopterygii (*Qiang Huo*), 6g, Radix Lateralis Praeparatus Aconiti

Carmichaeli (*Fu Zi*), 3g, stir-fried Fructus Crataegi (*Shan Zha*), 6g, Radix Angelicae Pubescentis (*Du Huo*), 6g, Radix Cyathulae (*Chuan Niu Xi*), 6g, Herba Ephedrae (*Ma Huang*), 3g, uncooked Cortex Phellodendri (*Huang Bai*), 9g, Radix Linderae Strychnifoliae (*Wu Yao*), 6g, dry Rhizoma Zingiberis (*Gan Jiang*), 3g, Semen Arecae Catechu (*Bing Lang*), 9g, Fructus Citri Aurantii (*Zhi Ke*), 3g, Radix Glycyrrhizae (*Gan Cao*), 3g, uncooked Rhizoma Coptidis Chinensis (*Huang Lian*), 6g, Fructus Gardeniae Jasminoidis (*Zhi Zi*), 9g

39
Atrophy of the Gums (*Ya Yin Wei Suo*)

This refers to gradual atrophy of the gums, possibly leading to exposure of the root of and loosening of teeth. It corresponds to receding gums in modern Western medicine.

Disease causes, disease mechanisms:

I. Stomach fire steaming upward

Addiction to alcohol, fatty, spicy, dry, and/or rich food may give rise to stomach fire. If this fire steams upward along the channel, it will burn and damage the network vessels and qi and blood in the gums, leading to consumption of the fluids and qi and blood. Therefore, the gums will receive less nourishment and become withered over time.

2. Kidney yin vacuity

Kidney yin vacuity may be due to aging, unrestrained sexual activity, or enduring disease. "The kidneys govern the bones", while the teeth are the surplus of the bones which depend on nourishment from kidney essence and marrow. If there is kidney yin vacuity, first, the teeth will become withered and soft. Secondly, yin vacuity fire will be engendered and flame upward, burning and damaging the network vessels and qi and blood of the gums. Over time, the gums will receive less and less nourishment, leading to withering of the gums and loose teeth.

3. Qi & blood vacuity

Constitutional vacuity or enduring disease may give rise to qi and blood vacuity. If there is blood vacuity, the gums cannot get sufficient nourishment. If there is qi vacuity, there will be bleeding due to poor containment of the blood by the qi. Therefore, there will be withered gums accompanied by bleeding between the teeth.

Treatment based on pattern discrimination:

1. Stomach fire steaming upward

Symptoms: Withered gums following red, swollen gums with discharge of blood and pus, exposure of the roots of the teeth, vexatious thirst and a liking for chilled drinks, increased food intake but easy hungering, a clamoring stomach, constipation, dark-colored urine, a red crimson tongue with yellow, thick fur, and a surging, large or slippery, rapid pulse

Therapeutic principles: Clear the stomach and drain fire, disperse swelling and stop pain

Acupuncture & moxibustion:

Di Cang (St 4)	Unblocks the channel and clears heat to stop pain. Direct the tip of the needle first to *Ying Xiang* (LI 20) and then to *Cheng Jiang* (CV 24).
Pi Shu (Bl 20) *Wei Shu* (Bl 21)	Together, these points nourish the stomach and clear heat therein.
Nei Ting (St 44) *Fu Liu* (Ki 7)	Together, these points clear stomach heat and nourish stomach yin.

Additions & subtractions: For constipation, add *Tian Shu* (St 25). For toothache in the upper teeth, add *Jiao Sun* (TB 20), while for toothache in the lower teeth, add *Da Ying* (St 5). For vexation and insomnia, add *Nei Guan* (Per 6).

Chinese medicinal formula: Modified *Qing Wei San* (Clear the Stomach Powder)

Ingredients: Uncooked Gypsum Fibrosum (*Shi Gao*), 18g, wine stir-fried Rhizoma Coptidis Chinensis (*Huang Lian*), 6g, uncooked Radix Rehmanniae (*Sheng Di*), 15g, uncooked Radix Angelicae Sinensis (*Dang Gui*), 9g, Cortex Radicis Moutan (*Dan Pi*), 9g, uncooked Rhizoma Cimicifugae (*Sheng Ma*), 3g, Radix Glycyrrhizae (*Gan Cao*), 3g, Fructus Gardeniae Jasminoidis (*Zhi Zi*), 9g, uncooked Radix Et Rhizoma Rhei (*Da Huang*), 6g, Radix Scrophulariae Ningpoensis (*Xuan Shen*), 9g

2. Kidney yin vacuity

Symptoms: Withered gums with erosion that bleeds, loose teeth, exposure of the roots of the teeth, dizziness, tinnitus, pain and weakness of the low back and knees, a sensation of heat in the palms of the hands and soles of the feet, a slightly red tongue with reduced fur, and a fine, rapid pulse

Therapeutic principles: Enrich yin and supplement the kidneys, boost the essence and secure the teeth

Acupuncture & moxibustion:

Da Ying (St 5)   Quickens the network vessels

Guan Yuan (CV 4)   Together, these points enrich yin and boost the
San Yin Jiao (Sp 6)   essence to secure the teeth.
Tai Xi (Ki 3)

Or use *Pi Shu* (Bl 20), *Ge Shu* (Bl 17), *Shen Shu* (Bl 23) and *Guan Yuan Shu* (Bl 26) instead.

Additions & subtractions: For seminal emission, add *Zhi Shi* (Bl 52). For sore throat, add *Zhao Hai* (Ki 6).

Chinese medicinal formula: Modified *Liu Wei Di Huang Wan* (Six Flavors Rehmannia Pills)

Ingredients: Prepared Radix Rehmanniae (*Shu Di*), 18g, steamed Fructus Corni Officinalis (*Shan Zhu Yu*), 12g, stir-fried Radix Dioscoreae Oppositae (*Shan Yao*), 9g, Sclerotium Poriae Cocos (*Fu Ling*), 6g, Cortex Radicis Moutan (*Dan Pi*), 6g, Rhizoma Alismatis (*Ze Xie*), 6g, Rhizoma Drynariae (*Gu Sui Bu*), 9g, salt stir-fried Radix Achyranthis Bidentatae (*Niu Xi*), 9g, Radix Dipsaci (*Xu Duan*), 9g, Fructus Lycii Chinensis (*Gou Qi Zi*), 9g

3. Qi & blood vacuity

Symptoms: Withered gums which are pale white in color, exposure of the roots of the teeth, forceless chewing, bleeding from between the teeth, especially when brushing the teeth, fear of cold, fatigue, dizziness, flowery (*i.e.*, blurred) vision, insomnia, profuse dreaming during sleep, heart palpitations and racing heart, shortage of qi with disinclination to speak, a pale tongue with thin, white fur, and a deep, fine pulse

Therapeutic principles: Supplement the blood and boost the qi, nourish the gums and fortify the teeth

Acupuncture & moxibustion:

He Gu (LI 4)	Together, these points supplement the qi.
Zu San Li (St 36)	

San Yin Jiao (Sp 6)	Together, these points fortify the spleen to
Pi Shu (Bl 20)	engender and nourish the blood.
Ge Shu (Bl 17)	

Additions & subtractions: For severe heart palpitations and racing heart, add *Shen Men* (Ht 7) and *Nei Guan* (Per 6). For poor appetite, add *Jian Li* (CV 11).

Chinese medicinal formula: Modified *Ba Zhen Tang* (Eight Pearls Decoction)

Ingredients: Prepared Radix Rehmanniae (*Shu Di*), 12g, Radix Angelicae Sinensis (*Dang Gui*), 9g, Radix Albus Paeoniae Lactiflorae (*Bai Shao*), 15g, uncooked Radix Ligustici Wallichii (*Chuan Xiong*), 6g, honey stir-fried Radix Codonopsitis Pilosulae (*Dang Shen*), 9g, bran stir-fried Rhizoma Atractylodis Macrocephalae (*Bai Zhu*), 9g, Sclerotium Poriae Cocos (*Fu Ling*), 9g, mix-fried Radix Glycyrrhizae (*Zhi Gan Cao*), 6g, Rhizoma Drynariae (*Gu Sui Bu*), 9g, salt stir-fried Radix Achyranthis Bidentatae (*Niu Xi*), 9g

40
Bleeding Gums (*Ya Yin Chu Xue*)

This refers to bleeding from between the teeth or from between the teeth and gums.

Disease causes, disease mechanisms:

I. Exuberant stomach fire

Addiction to spicy food may lead to heat accumulating in the stomach. If this heat transforms into fire and flames upward along the channel to the gums, burning and damaging the network vessels in the gums, there will be bleeding gums.

2. Yin vacuity fire of the stomach

Constitutional stomach yin vacuity is often the cause of yin vacuity fire of the stomach. If this fire flames upward along the channel to the gums, burning and damaging the network vessels there, bleeding gums will occur.

3. Liver-kidney yin vacuity

Yin vacuity of the liver and kidneys is often due to constitutional kidney yin vacuity, enduring disease, unrestrained sexual activity, or aging. Yin is supposed to check yang. If yin is vacuous, yin cannot check yang efficiently, thus giving rise to yin vacuity fire. If this fire flames upward, burning and damaging the network vessels in the gums, there will be bleeding gums.

4. Spleen vacuity not containing the blood

Both dietary irregularities and taxation can result in the spleen becoming vacuous. This then leads to central qi vacuity. Central qi is responsible for containing and restraining the blood within its vessels. Being vacuous, the spleen qi cannot contain the blood, and this may give rise to bleeding gums.

Treatment based on discrimination:

I. Exuberant stomach fire

Symptoms: Bleeding gums with profuse, bright red blood, red, swollen gums, bad breath, thirst with a desire to drink, constipation, a red tongue with yellow fur, and a slippery, rapid pulse

Therapeutic principles: Clear heat and drain fire, cool the blood and stop bleeding

Acupuncture & moxibustion:

San Jian (LI 3) *Shang Yang* (LI 1)	Together, these points clear heat in the *yang ming* when pricked to bleed.
Chong Yang (St 42) *Nei Ting* (St 44)	Together, these points clear and drain stomach fire to stop bleeding.
Wei Zhong (Bl 40)	Cools the blood to stop bleeding when pricked to bleed

Additions & subtractions: For constipation, add *Tian Shu* (St 25). For profuse dreaming, add *Li Dui* (St 45).

Chinese medicinal formula: Modified *Qing Wei San* (Clear the Stomach Powder)

Ingredients: Uncooked Gypsum Fibrosum (*Shi Gao*), 30g, wine stir-fried Radix Scutellariae Baicalensis (*Huang Qin*), 9g, wine stir-fried Rhizoma Coptidis Chinensis (*Huang Lian*), 6g, uncooked Radix Rehmanniae (*Sheng Di*), 20g, Cortex Radicis Moutan (*Dan Pi*), 6g, uncooked Rhizoma Cimicifugae (*Sheng Ma*), 3g, Fructus Gardeniae Jasminoidis (*Zhi Zi*), 9g

Additions & subtractions: If the constipation is severe, add uncooked Radix Et Rhizoma Rhei (*Da Huang*), 6g, and Mirabilitum (*Mang Xiao*), 6g. If there is concomitant kidney yin vacuity, subtract uncooked Radix Rehmanniae (*Sheng Di*) and Fructus Gardeniae Jasminoidis (*Zhi Zi*) and add prepared Radix Rehmanniae (*Shu Di*), 15g, Tuber Ophiopogonis Japonici (*Mai Men Dong*), 9g, salt mix-fried Rhizoma Anemarrhenae Asphodeloidis (*Zhi Mu*), 9g, and salt stir-fried Radix Achyranthis Bidentatae (*Niu Xi*), 9g.

2. Yin vacuity fire of the stomach

Symptoms: Bleeding gums with pale red blood, gum erosion, slightly painful, swollen gums, a red tongue with thin, dry fur and reduced moisture, and a slippery, rapid, forceless pulse

Therapeutic principles: Clear the stomach and nourish yin

Acupuncture & moxibustion:

Ge Shu (Bl 17)	Together, these points nourish yin blood and help
Pi Shu (Bl 20)	clear the stomach to stop bleeding.
Wei Shu (Bl 21)	
Nei Ting (St 44)	Together, these points nourish yin and clear the
Fu Liu (Ki 7)	stomach to stop bleeding.

Chinese medicinal formula: Modified *Yu Nu Jian* (Jade Maiden Decoction)

Ingredients: Uncooked Gypsum Fibrosum (*Shi Gao*), 18g, prepared Radix Rehmanniae (*Shu Di*), 18g, salt mix-fried Rhizoma Anemarrhenae Asphodeloidis (*Zhi Mu*), 9g, salt mix-fried Cortex Phellodendri (*Huang Bai*), 9g, salt stir-fried Radix Achyranthis Bidentatae (*Niu Xi*), 9g, Tuber Ophiopogonis Japonici (*Mai Men Dong*), 9g, Herba Dendrobii (*Shi Hu*), 9g

3. Liver-kidney yin vacuity

Symptoms: Bleeding gums with scanty, pale red blood, loose teeth, dizziness, tinnitus, pain and weakness of the low back and knees, a tender, red tongue with reduced fur, and a fine, rapid pulse

Therapeutic principles: Enrich yin, downbear fire, and stop bleeding

Acupuncture and moxibustion:

Ge Shu (Bl 17)	Together, these points nourish the blood to
Pi Shu (Bl 20)	engender the essence.
Wei Shu (Bl 21)	
Shen Shu (Bl 23)	Together, these points enrich yin, downbear fire,
Tai Xi (Ki 3)	and stop bleeding.
San Yin Jiao (Sp 6)	

Chinese medicinal formula: Modified *Zhi Bai Di Huang Wan* (Anemarrhena & Phellodendron Rehmannia Pills)

Ingredients: Prepared Radix Rehmanniae (*Shu Di*), 18g, steamed Fructus Corni Officinalis (*Shan Zhu Yu*), 9g, Sclerotium Poriae Cocos (*Fu Ling*), 6g, salt mix-fried Rhizoma Alismatis (*Ze Xie*), 6g, Cortex Radicis Moutan (*Dan Pi*), 12g, salt mix-fried Rhizoma Anemarrhenae Asphodeloidis (*Zhi Mu*), 9g, salt mix-fried Cortex Phellodendri (*Huang Bai*), 9g, Cortex Radicis Lycii Chinensis (*Di Gu Pi*), 9g, salt stir-fried Radix Achyranthis Bidentatae (*Niu Xi*), 9g, Rhizoma Drynariae (*Gu Sui Bu*), 9g

4. Spleen vacuity not containing the blood

Symptoms: Bleeding gums on slight stimulation, blood possibly profuse in amount, bleeding worse when fatigued, pale gums, easy bruising due to relatively slight pressure, fatigued spirit and lack of strength, a low, timorous voice, a bright white or sallow yellow facial complexion, a fat, pale tongue with thin, white fur, and a fine, weak pulse

Therapeutic principles: Fortify the spleen, boost the qi, and contain the blood

Acupuncture & moxibustion:

Ge Shu (Bl 17)	Together, these points fortify the spleen and
Pi Shu (Bl 20)	stomach to promote the engendering of qi and
Wei Shu (Bl 21)	blood when needled with supplementing method.
Zu San Li (St 36)	Together, these points boost the qi and contain the
He Gu (LI 4)	blood to stop bleeding when needled with supplementing method.

Chinese medicinal formula: Modified *Gui Pi Tang* (Return the Spleen Decoction)

Ingredients: Honey stir-fried Radix Astragali Membranacei (*Huang Qi*), 20g, bran stir-fried Rhizoma Atractylodis Macrocephalae (*Bai Zhu*), 9g, stir-fried Radix Angelicae Sinensis (*Dang Gui*), 6g, Sclerotium Poriae Cocos (*Fu Ling*), 9g, Radix Auklandiae Lappae (*Mu Xiang*), 6g, mix-fried Radix Glycyrrhizae (*Zhi Gan Cao*), 6g, Radix Codonopsitis Pilosulae (*Dang Shen*), 15g, Arillus Euphoriae Longanae (*Long Yan Rou*), 9g, stir-fried Semen Zizyphi Spinosae (*Suan Zao Ren*), 9g, Herba Agrimoniae Pilosae (*Xian He Cao*), 9g, Rhizoma Bletillae Striatae (*Bai Ji*), 9g, Cacumen Biotae Orientalis (*Ce Bai Ye*), 9g

Note: Bleeding gums are a relatively commonly encountered symptom in Western clinical practice. Very commonly, there is a combination of heat in the stomach forcing the blood to move recklessly outside its pathways and spleen qi vacuity not containing the blood within its vessels. In young and middle-aged adults, this stomach heat is due to liver depression transforming heat and is then aggravated by either stress, alcohol, or spicy, acrid, pepper, and/or fatty food. The spleen vacuity is then aggravated by fatigue and over-taxation. As middle-aged patients age, this scenario may be further complicated by stomach yin vacuity and/or liver-kidney vacuity.

Besides acupuncture and Chinese medicinals taken internally, it is very important to modify the diet, avoiding heat-engendering foods as well as spleen-weakening ones. Careful brushing of the teeth *and* gums and daily massage of the gums by tapping with the fingertips are also important to maintain the health of the gums and teeth. For further information on self-massage of the teeth and gums, see Fan Ya-li's *Chinese Self-massage Therapy, The Easy Way to Health* also published by Blue Poppy Press.

Bibliography

Chinese language:

Lin Chuang Bi Du (Clinical Obligatory Readings) by Ou Yang-qi, China Chinese Medicine Press, Beijing, 1993

Lin Chuang Bian Zheng Shi Zhi Xue (A Study of the Clinical Basing of Treatment on Pattern Discrimination) by Liu Bin, Science, Technology & Literature Press, Beijing, 1992

Shi Yong Zhong Yi Zhen Duan Xue (A Study of Practical Chinese Medicine Diagnosis) by Liu Tie-tiao, Shanghai Science & Technology Press, Shanghai, 1988

Zhong Yi Bing Yin Bing Ji Xue (A Study of Chinese Medicine Disease Causes & Disease Mechanisms) by Song Lu-bing, People's Health & Hygiene Press, Beijing, 1987

Zhong Yi Da Ci Dian, Nei Ke Fen Ce (Encyclopedia of Chinese Medicine, Volume on Internal Medicine), People's Health & Hygiene Press, Beijing, 1987

Zhong Yi Nei Ke Xue (A Study of Chinese Medicine Internal Medicine) by Zhang Bo-Yu, People's Health & Hygiene Press, Beijing, 1988

Zhong Yi Nei Ke Zheng Zhuang Bian Zhi Shou Ce (A Handbook of Chinese Medicine Internal Medicine Symptoms Discrimination & Treatment) by Fang Wen-xian, Liu Qing & Chu Xiu-jun, China Standard Press, Beijing, 1989

Zhong Yi Zheng Hou Zhen Duan Zhi Liao Xue (A Study of Chinese Medicine Patterns, Diagnosis & Treatment) by Cheng Shao-en & Xia Hong-sheng, Beijing Science & Technology Press, Beijing, 1993

Zhong Yi Zheng Zhuang Jian Bie Zhen Duan Xue (A Study of Chinese Medicine Symptoms & Differential Diagnosis) by Zhao Jin-ze, People's Health & Hygiene Press, Beijing, 1984

Zhong Yi Zhi Liao Xue (A Study of Chinese Medicine Treatments) by Sun Guo-jie & Tu Jin-wen, China Medicine & Medicinals Science & Technology Press, Beijing, 1990

English language:

Chinese Acupuncture & Moxibustion edited by Cheng Xin-nong, Foreign Languages Press, Beijing, 1987

Chinese Herbal Medicine: Formulas & Strategies by Dan Bensky & Randall Barolet, Eastland Press, Seattle, 1990

Chinese Herbal Medicine: Materia Medica by Dan Bensky & Andrew Gamble, Eastland Press, Seattle, 1993

Fundamentals of Chinese Acupuncture by Andrew Ellis, Nigel Wiseman & Ken Boss, Paradigm Publications, Brookline, MA, 1988

Fundamentals of Chinese Medicine translated & amended by Nigel Wiseman & Andrew Ellis, Paradigm Publications, Brookline, MA, 1985

Glossary of Chinese Medical Terms and Acupuncture Points by Nigel Wiseman, Paradigm Publications, Brookline, MA, 1990

Pao Zhi: An Introduction to the Use of Processed Chinese Medicinals by Philippe Sionneau, Blue Poppy Press, Boulder, CO, 1995

Seventy Essential TCM Formulas for Beginners by Bob Flaws, Blue Poppy Press, Boulder, CO, 1994

Statements of Fact in TCM by Bob Flaws, Blue Poppy Press, Boulder, CO, 1994

Other books by Philippe Sionneau

L'Acupuncture Pratiquée en Chine, Tome I: Les Points Traditionels, Guy Trédaniel Editeur, Paris, 1994

L'Acupuncture Pratiquée en Chine, Tome II: Les Traitements Efficaces, Guy Trédaniel Editeur, Paris, 1994

Pao Zhi: An Introduction to the Use of Processed Chinese Medicinals, translated by Bob Flaws, Blue Poppy Press, Boulder, CO, 1994

Pharmacopée Chinoise et Acupuncture: Les Prescriptions Efficaces. Guy Trédaniel Editeur, Paris, 1996

Pharmacopée Chinoise: L'Art des Associations en Pratique. Guy Trédaniel Editeur, Paris (forthcoming in 1997)

Toubles Psychiques en médecine Chinoise: Les Solutions de L'Acupuncture et de la Pharmacopée Chinoise. Guy Trédaniel Editeur, Paris

Troubles Psychologiques et Psychiatriques en Médecine Chinoise, Editions Rouergue, forthcoming in 1996

Utilization Clinique de la Pharmocopée Chinoise, Tome 1: Les Substances Médicinales Preparée, So Dai Editions, Paris, 1994

Utilization Clinique de la Pharmacopée Chinoise, Tome 2: Traitment Efficaces: Selection des Substances Médicinales-cles, Editions Rouergue, forthcoming in 1996

Formula Index

A, B

An Gong Niu Huang Wan 120, 147
Ba Zhen Tang 108, 194, 223
Bai Hu Jia Ren Shen Tang 150
Bai Hu Tang 40, 96
Ban Xia Bai Zhu Tian Ma Tang 124
Bao He Wan 18, 32, 192
Bu Zhong Yi Qi Tang 51, 167, 178, 204

C, D

Can Shi Tang 52
Chai Hu Qing Gan Yin 16
Chai Hu Shu Gan San 35
Da Cheng Qi Tang 41, 154
Da Xian Xiong Tang 50
Dang Gui Long Hui Wan 159
Dao Chi San 136, 158, 165
Dao Tan Tang 124
Di Tan Tang 118, 132
Ding Xian Wan 56, 119

E, F, G

Er Chen Tang 14
Er Jia Fu Mai Tang 186
Fang Feng Tong Sheng San 92
Gan Cao Gan Jiang Tang 68
Gan Lu Xiao Du Dan 29
Ge Hua Jie Cheng Tang 112
Gua Lou Xie Bai Ban Xia Tang 76
Gui Pi Tang 77, 82, 109, 129, 161, 229

H

Huan Shao Dan 181
Huang Lian Jie Du Tang 45, 141, 158
Huang Lian Shang Qing Wan 199
Huo Luo Liu Qi Yin 217
Huo Po Xia Ling Tang 4

J, K, L, M

Jia Wei Fu Mai Tang 130
Jin Fo Cao San 199
Kou Chuang San 64
Leng Xiao Wan 75
Li Zhong Wan 67
Liang Ge San 62, 86, 99, 166
Ling Yang Jiao Gou Teng Tang 110, 146
Liu Jun Zi Tang 2, 17, 59, 83, 104
Liu Wei Di Huang Wan 143, 182, 222
Long Dan Xie Gan Tang 9, 137
Ma Huang Fu Zi Xi Xin Tang 200
Ma Xing Shi Gan Tang 39, 73
Meng Shi Gun Tan Wan 140

P, Q

Ping Wei San 3, 28
Qi Wei Bai Zhu San 25
Qian Zheng San 55, 116
Qing Qi Hua Tan Wan 30, 74, 125
Qing Shu Yi Qi Tang 43
Qing Wei San 33, 87, 138, 173, 181, 191,
    202, 221, 226
Qing Wei Tang 210, 215
Qing Xin Liang Ge San 99
Qing Ying Tang 42
Qing Zao Jiu Fei Tang 44, 131

S, T

San Jia Fu Mai Tang 111
Shen Ling Bai Zhu San 101
Shen Qi Wan 13, 169
Shi Xiao San 76
Si Jun Zi Tang 94
Si Ni Tang 79
Si Wu Tang 122, 168
Si Wu Xiao Feng Yin 93
Tian Ma Gou Teng Yin 57

Tian Wang Bu Xin Dan 142
Tiao Wei Cheng Qi Tang 93, 96
Tong Qiao Huo Xue Tang 51
Tuo Li Xiao Du San 211

W, X

Wei Jing Tang 34
Wei Rui Tang 47
Wu Ling San 48
Wu Mei Wan 60, 193
Wu Wei Xiao Du Yin 209
Xi Jiao Di Huang Tang 43, 216
Xiang Sha Liu Jun Zi Tang 2, 83
Xiao Chai Hu Tang 8, 10
Xiao Yao San 10, 77, 177
Xie Bai San 22, 139
Xie Huang San 24, 58, 100
Xie Huang Tang 70
Xie Xin Tang 131, 176

Y, Z

Yin Qiao San 39
Yu Nu Jian 187, 227
Yu Ye Tang 47
Zeng Ye Tang 151, 155
Zhen Gan Xi Feng Tang 111, 123, 195
Zhen Wu Tang 66, 105, 152
Zhi Bai Di Huang Wan 12, 46, 63, 160,
    168, 174, 203, 228
Zhi Zi Da Huang Tang 100
Zhu Ling Tang 49
Zi Chun Yin 89
Zi Yin Di Huang Wan 88

General Index

A

abdomen, distention and fullness in the stomach and 28
abdominal distention 2, 17, 94, 101
abdominal distention and fullness which is worse after eating 101
abdominal pain, intermittent 192
abdominal pain that refuses pressure 40
addictions to peculiar foods 192
AIDS 170
alcohol addiction, history of 112
allergies, chronic 170
amenorrhea 82
anxiety and agitation 100
appetite, poor 2, 3, 8, 17, 28, 52, 58, 66, 94, 138, 177, 214, 223
appetite, reduced 1, 3
asthma 39, 65, 156
auditory acuity, reduced 181
autoimmune diseases 170

B

bag-over-the-head sensation 13
belching and burping 35
belching, putrid 17, 32
belching, sour 17
bleeding from the tongue, persistent 158, 159
bleeding of the tongue, spontaneous 157
bleeding, spontaneous external 86
blood ejection 42, 44, 86
body aches 98, 217
borborygmus 48, 49
breath, bad 29, 31-35, 57, 87, 96, 138, 165, 173, 180, 190, 201, 210, 214, 217, 226
breath, bad, with sour smell 32
breath, shortness of 2, 46, 66
breath, shortness of exacerbated on exertion 66
breath sometimes smelling fishy 21
breathing, rapid 21, 73
bruxism 189, 190, 195

C

cancer 170
CFIDS 170
cheekbones, red 88, 129, 146, 160
cheeks, swollen 61
chest and lateral costal region, glomus and fullness in the 4
chest and lateral costal regions, pain and fullness in the 16
chest, fullness and stabbing pain in the 75
chest, fullness in the 4, 8, 16, 74, 140, 145
chest oppression and lateral costal distention 35
chest, pain and distention in the 34
chest pain radiating to upper back 75-76
chest, vexation and pain in the 43
chew food, inability to 199
chewing, difficulty 181
chewing, forceless 222
cholecystitis 10
clouding collapse 110, 117, 118
cold, aversion to 4, 98, 200, 208
cold environment, preference for 100
cold, fear of 12, 78, 222
coma 117-119, 147
constipation 16, 18, 24, 25, 32-33, 40, 49, 57, 62, 69, 86-88, 92, 93, 95, 100, 125, 131, 137-140, 146, 154, 159, 165, 172, 173, 180, 186, 191, 201, 206, 210, 214, 220, 226, 227
convulsions 67, 109, 118, 194
cough 21, 22, 29, 34, 39, 44, 49, 65, 73-76, 125, 131, 139
cough and panting 73
cough and panting with expectoration 75
cough and panting with phlegm rales 74
cough with expectoration of thick, yellow phlegm 125
cough with foamy expectoration 49
cough with no phlegm, dry 44
cough with rapid breathing, dry 73
cough with thick, yellow phlegm 29

cough with yellow phlegm which is difficult to expectorate 73
crab-claw markings 51

D

deafness 111, 129, 159
defecation, inhibited 52, 100, 105, 191
defecation, uneasy 93, 131
delirium 41, 42, 119, 154, 158
delirium, clouded spirit and 41
diarrhea 3, 18, 32, 38, 52, 58, 67, 98, 191
diarrhea, chronic 3
diarrhea, sloppy 58
diarrhea with abdominal pain 191
digestion, swift with rapid hungering 190
dizziness 8, 9, 12, 45-47, 55, 66, 82, 83, 92, 101, 108, 109, 123-125, 132, 137, 159, 160, 167, 181, 182, 193, 202, 203, 221, 222, 228
dreaming, profuse 12, 108, 110, 141, 158, 222, 226
drool, expectoration of foamy 83
drooling, foamy 118
drooling of clear, thin saliva 58
drooling, persistent 55
dysmenorrhea 51
dyspnea 74

E

eating, no pleasure in 2
edema in the face 48
edema of the eyelids and face 49
edema, puffy 152, 217
emaciation 59, 155, 160, 192
emotional disturbance, recent history of 177
enuresis 68
epistaxis 86
eyelids and face, edema of the 50
eyes, deviated mouth and 54-56, 116, 124
eyes, inability to close the 54
eyes, painful, distended 123
eyes, red 40, 137
eyes, red face and 8, 16, 159

F

face, edema in the 48
face, eyes, red 9, 17, 165
face, tidal flushing of the 150
facial complexion, bright, white 50, 58
facial complexion, dull, yellow 59
facial complexion, pale yellow 101
facial complexion, sallow 192
facial complexion, soot black 51
facial complexion, white, lusterless 74, 128
facial complexion, withered yellow 77, 82
facial numbness 54
fatigue 4, 12, 17, 27, 43, 46, 50, 66, 83, 94, 104, 108, 111, 122, 152, 161, 167, 178, 203, 222, 230
feet, heat in the palms of the hands and soles of the 151, 221
feet, sensation of heat in the hands and 167
feet, tingling and numbness in the hands and 108
fever 4, 8, 22, 34, 39-41, 43-45, 47-50, 55, 73, 86, 88, 98, 109, 111, 119, 120, 129, 130, 146, 147, 150, 154, 160, 166, 172, 182, 199, 208, 214-216
fever and chills, alternating 8
fever and chills, intermittent 214, 215
fever, great 40, 44
fever, high 4, 45, 47, 119, 146, 147, 150, 215, 216
fever in the afternoon, tidal 49
fever, low 129, 130, 166
fever, steaming bone tidal 45
fever, tidal 45, 49, 88, 120, 154, 160, 182
fever, unresolved 73
fever which is worse at night 111
fever with either no or inhibited sweating 39
fever worse at night 41, 150
flatulence with foul smell 32
food intake large, rapid hungering 24

G

genital swelling 9

glomus and oppression in the chest and abdomen 3, 53, 79, 138, 197
glomus in the stomach and abdomen 41
gum erosion 227
gum, painful swelling of, with fissuring 211
gums, abscess in the 209
gums, atrophy of the 219
gums, bleeding 225-230
gums, distended, swollen 198, 217
gums, gaping 180, 182
gums, pain & swelling of the 207
gums, painful, swollen 33, 138, 197, 207, 208, 211, 214, 227
gums, putrefying 213
gums, red, hard, painful, swollen 208
gums, withered 220-222

H

hair loss 182, 187
hands, heat in the palms of the. and soles of the feet 151, 167, 222
head, distention and pain in the 109
head, feeling of a tight band around the 13
headache 8, 9, 39, 44, 44, 56, 83, 123, 159, 199, 202, 203, 205, 208, 214
heart and abdomen, hardness and fullness between the 49
heart palpitations 66, 77, 78, 82, 98, 108, 122, 128, 132, 141, 193, 202, 203, 222, 223
heart, racing 77, 108, 128, 129, 141, 222, 223
heart, vexatious heat in the 47, 158
hearts, vexatious heat in the five 12, 45, 63, 141, 155, 160, 173, 194
hemiplegia 55-56, 116, 118
hiccup 89
hunger without desire for food 89
hungering, easy 57, 165, 220
hungering, large food intake with rapid 24
hungering, swift digestion with rapid 190

I, J

insomnia 30, 44-46, 49, 63, 77, 78, 82, 88, 93, 104, 108, 110, 112, 122, 128, 140-142, 155, 158, 186, 191, 195, 202, 221, 222
irascibility 89, 16, 137, 159
irritability 35
itching, pudendal 9
jaundice 10
jaw, clenched 117

L

lacrimation 54
lassitude with no willingness to move 100
lateral costal region, burning pain in the 159
lateral costal region, pain exacerbated by coughing 48
lie flat, inability to 74, 75
limbs, cumbersome 13
limbs, encumbered 48, 49, 101, 132, 140
limbs, fatigued 128, 166
limbs lacking warmth 12, 78, 104, 152, 169
limbs, numb 123, 124
limbs, trembling and hypertonic 110
limbs, trembling 111, 112
limbs, weakness of the 50
lip tremor 91, 92
lips, blue 132, 145
lips, cracked dry 85
lips, crimson 69
lips, cyanotic 71-78
lips, dry 57, 85, 87-89, 93, 172
lips, pale white 81, 128
lips, quivering, itchy, dry 93
lips, red, swollen, cracked, dry 87
lips, red, swollen, itching 92
lips, restless licking of the 57
lips, translucent milliary eruptions on the inside of the 192
low back and knee soreness and weakness 78
low back and spine, pain and weakness of the 202

M

macules and papules, faintly visible 41
macules, eruption of 44
macules, purple or black 42
mania 42
meat stagnation 18
memory, impaired 77, 108, 122, 128, 160
menstruation, delayed 82
menstruation, scanty 108
menstruation with purple, black clots 51
mouth, acrid taste in the 21, 22, 139
mouth and tongue, sores in the with
    frequent recurrence 67
mouth, bland taste in the 1, 2, 18, 27, 98
mouth, bitter taste in the 7-10, 29, 99,
    125, 136, 137, 140, 159, 173, 210, 217
mouth, drooling from the corner of the
    53, 54
mouth, dry, and throat 12, 142, 150, 160,
    194
mouth, dry, with desire to drink 24
mouth, dry, with no desire to drink 25,
    34, 167
mouth, gaping 73
mouth, malodorous 31, 33
mouth, peppery taste in the 21
mouth, salty taste in the 11-12
mouth, sliminess in the 3, 4, 13, 27-30, 67
mouth sores 54, 57, 61, 63, 64, 69, 86
mouth, sores in the, bright red 61
mouth, sour and bitter tastes in the 16
mouth, sour taste in the 15-19, 31
mouth, sweet taste in the 5, 23-26

N

nails, lusterless 82
nails, pale white lips and 128
nausea 3, 132, 214
navel, pain around the 59
night sweats 45, 63, 88, 130, 142, 160,
    182, 194
nose and throat, dry 44
nosebleed 42, 44
nostrils, flaring 73

nostrils, itching in the 192

P, R

palms and skin, burning heat in the 100
palpitations around the umbilicus 71
panting and cough with expectoration 81
panting on exertion 78
perspiration, spontaneous 161, 178, 203
phlegm, profuse 112
posture, curled-up lying 105
restlessness 99
roundworm macules of white color 192
roundworms 59, 60, 189, 190, 192-193

S

saliva, excessive 5, 65
scanty or no sweating 48
scrotum, shrinking of the 145
seminal emission 88, 143, 168, 180, 222
shoulders, raised 73
sighing, frequent 17, 76, 177
skin, burning heat in the palms and 100
skin, scaly 51
sleep at night, disquieted 164
sleep, reduced 12, 41, 160
sleep, vexation with reduced 41
somnolence 104, 129
speak, disinclination to 12, 50, 66, 77,
    161, 166, 178, 193, 203, 222
speech, confused 44
speech, inhibited 55, 56, 116, 123, 132,
    140
spine, pain in the 202
spitting, frequent 65, 66, 68
spitting of foamy saliva, frequent 68
spirit, fatigued 68, 77, 129, 161, 181,
    191, 214, 229
spirit, lassitude of the 25, 105
steps, unsteady 110, 123
stomach and abdomen, fullness and
    oppression in the 2, 27, 67
stomach and abdomen, glomus in 40
stomach, burning in the 19
stomach, clamoring 87, 165, 190, 220

stomach, distention and oppression in the 17
stools, dry 16, 24, 49, 93, 130, 131
stools, loose 2, 3, 17, 27, 28, 50, 66, 83, 94, 101, 104, 152, 169, 181
stools, untransformed food in the 32
strength, lack of 2, 12, 17, 25, 27, 67, 68, 77, 83, 94, 101, 104, 108, 122, 152, 167, 178, 203, 229
sweating, great 40
sweating, scanty or no 47
sweating, spontaneous 50, 78, 178, 203
sweats, night 45, 63, 88, 130, 142, 160, 182, 194

T

teeth, blackening of the 185, 186
teeth, bleeding from between the 222, 225
teeth, distention and pain in the 198, 201
teeth, dull pain in the 202, 203
teeth, exposure of the roots of 220-222
teeth, falling of the 181
teeth, grinding the 189
teeth, grinding during sleep 191-192
teeth, loose 160, 179-182, 187, 202, 219, 221, 228
teeth, paroxysmal pain in, worsened by inhalation of cold air 200
thirst 21, 28, 29, 33, 37-52, 57, 62, 68, 73, 86, 87, 92, 95, 100, 112, 130, 131, 138-140, 150, 151, 154, 156, 158, 164, 165, 172, 173, 176, 180, 190, 199-201, 220, 226
thirst and dry throat which are worse at night 45
thirst, oral 37, 38
thirst, pseudo 37
thirst, severe 39-41
thirst, vexatious 57, 220
thirst with desire for warm drinks 50
thirst with liking for chilled drinks 33
throat, dry 8, 45, 131, 139, 186
throat, dry, sore 202
throat, gurgling sound of phlegm in the 55

throat, phlegm rales in the 56, 117, 215
throat, sore 39, 47, 86, 143, 168, 202, 222
tinnitus 12, 16, 45-47, 55, 56, 66, 123, 142, 159, 160, 168, 182, 193, 203, 221, 228
TMJ 195
tongue, bright red speckled eruptions on the tip of the 192
tongue, curled 145, 146
tongue, deviated 55, 116
tongue, dry 40, 41, 44, 48, 49, 130, 142, 149-151, 168, 201
tongue, dull, pale, swollen, with teeth-prints on 101
tongue, fat 78, 103-105, 203
tongue, fat, trembling 112
tongue, fissured 153-155
tongue, limp 127-129, 131, 132
tongue, numb, pale 122
tongue, numbness of the 121, 122, 126
tongue, obstinate, red sores on the 168
tongue, oozing of blood from the 160
tongue pain 24, 98, 141, 145
tongue, pain in the center of the 138
tongue, pain in the whole 140
tongue, pain, pricking, at the tip of the 136
tongue, pain, redness on the sides of the 137
tongue, painful, dry 142
tongue, pale, dry 151
tongue, pale, tender, fat, with teeth-prints 104, 105
tongue, persistent bleeding from 158-159
tongue, protracted 175-177
tongue, red, burning 141
tongue, red, limp, dry 130
tongue, red, numb, hypertonic 123
tongue, slight trembling of the 111
tongue sores 63, 69, 86, 1639, 16470
tongue, sores on the lips and 24
tongue, spontaneous bleeding of the 163
tongue, stiff 115-118, 172
tongue, stiff, crimson 119
tongue, swollen 97-101, 103, 158, 159
tongue, tingling sensation on the surface of the 21

tongue tip, red crimson 158
tongue, trembling 107, 110, 112
tongue, worrying 57, 171, 172
tooth decay 198, 204, 207, 209
tooth pain 197, 198, 205
torpid intake 13, 29, 76, 77

vomiting 3, 38, 48, 49, 52, 83, 89, 132,
    190, 214
vomiting, dry 89
vomiting of clear drool 49
vomiting of foamy drool 48
wind and cold, aversion to 39, 47, 54, 200

U

umbilicus, palpitations around the 66
urination frequent 12, 68, 169, 181
urination frequent and profuse 46
urination, frequent, at night 12, 181
urination, inhibited 48
urination, turbid dribbling 9
urine astringent voidings of dark-colored
    44, 158, 164
urine, clear 101, 152, 181, 217
urine, dark-colored 43, 44, 57, 73, 88,
    100, 125, 130, 131, 136, 139, 150,
    151, 158, 159, 176, 191, 201, 214, 220
urine, dribbling voidings of clear 181
urine, long voidings of clear 101
urine, reddish 28, 29
urine, short voidings of dark-colored 43,
    73, 100, 130, 131, 139, 150, 151
urine, short voidings of reddish 29
urine, short voidings of scant 13
urine, yellow 16, 21, 24, 33, 40, 49, 62,
    99

V, W

vaginal discharge, increased 9
veins, prominent 51
vertigo 8, 9, 16, 55, 56, 68, 110, 124,
    125, 132, 137, 159, 168, 181, 193
vexation 9, 16, 55, 68, 110, 124, 125,
    132, 137, 140, 145, 147, 150, 154,
    172, 176, 186, 190, 202, 221
vexation and agitation 16, 40, 44, 52, 99,
    109, 147, 150, 154, 172, 186
vexation a nd disquietude 29
vexation, vacuity 88, 202
voice, low while speaking 104, 128, 203

OTHER BOOKS ON CHINESE MEDICINE AVAILABLE FROM BLUE POPPY PRESS

1775 Linden Ave, Boulder, CO 80304
For ordering 1-800-487-9296
PH. 303\447-8372 FAX 303\447-0740

A NEW AMERICAN ACUPUNCTURE by Mark Seem, ISBN 0-936185-44-9, $22.95

ACUPUNCTURE AND MOXI-BUSTION FORMULAS & TREATMENTS by Cheng Dan-an, trans. By Wu Ming, ISBN 0-936185-68-6, $22.95

ACUTE ABDOMINAL SYN-DROMES: Their Diagnosis & Treatment by Combined Chinese-Western Medicine by Alon Marcus, ISBN 0-936185-31-7, $16.95

AGING & BLOOD STASIS: A New Approach to TCM Geriatrics, by Yan De-xin, ISBN 0-936185-63-5, $21.95

AIDS & ITS TREATMENT ACCORDING TO TRADITIONAL CHINESE MEDICINE by Huang Bing-shan, trans. by Fu-Di & Bob Flaws, ISBN 0-936185-28-7 $25.95

ARISAL OF THE CLEAR: A Simple Guide to Healthy Eating According to Traditional Chinese Medicine by Bob Flaws, ISBN #-936185-27-9 $10.95

THE BOOK OF JOOK: Chinese Medicinal Porridges, An Alternative to the Typical Western Breakfast, by Bob Flaws,

ISBN0-936185-60-0, $16.95

THE BREAST CONNECTION: A Laywoman's Guide to the Treatment of Breast Disease by Chinese Medicine by Honora Lee Wolfe ISBN 0-936185-61-9, $10.95

CHINESE MEDICAL PALMIS-TRY: Your Health in Your Hand, by Zong Xiao-fan & Gary Liscum, ISBN 0-936185-64-3, $15.95

CHINESE MEDICINAL TEAS: Simple, Proven, Folk Formulas for Common Diseases & Promoting Health, by Zong Xiao-fan & Gary Liscum, ISBN 0-936185-76-7, $19.95

CHINESE MEDICINAL WINES & ELIXIRS by Bob Flaws, ISBN 0-936185-58-9, $18.95

CHINESE PEDIATRIC MAS-SAGE THERAPY: A Parent's & Practitioner's Guide to the Prevention & Treatment of Childhood Illness, by Fan Ya-li, ISBN 0-936185-54-6, $12.95

CHINESE SELF-MASSAGE THERAPY: The Easy Way to Health, by Fan Ya-li ISBN 0-936185-74-0, $15.95

CLASSICAL MOXIBUSTION SKILLS in Contemporary Clinical Practice by Sung Baek, ISBN 0-936185-16-3 $12.95

A COMPENDIUM OF TCM PATTERNS & TREATMENTS by Bob Flaws & Daniel Finney, ISBN 0-936185-70-8, $29.95

THE DAO OF INCREASING LONGEVITY AND CONSERVING ONE'S LIFE by Anna Lin & Bob Flaws, ISBN 0-936185-24-4 $16.95

THE DIVINELY RESPONDING CLASSIC: A Translation of the *Shen Ying Jing* from *Zhen Jiu Da Cheng*, trans. by Yang Shou-zhong & Liu Feng-ting ISBN 0-936185-55-4, $15.95

ENDOMETRIOSIS, INFERTILITY AND TRADITIONAL CHINESE MEDICINE: A Laywoman's Guide by Bob Flaws ISBN 0-936185-14-7 $10.95

EXTRA TREATISES BASED ON INVESTIGATION & INQUIRY: A Translation of Zhu Dan-xi's *Ge Zhi Yu Lun*, by Yang Shou-zhong & Duan Wu-jin, ISBN 0-936185-53-8, $15.95

FIRE IN THE VALLEY: The TCM Diagnosis and Treatment of Vaginal Diseases by Bob Flaws ISBN 0-936185-25-2 $17.95

FLESHING OUT THE BONES: The Importance of Case Histories in Chin. Med. trans. by Chip Chace. ISBN 0-936185-30-9, $18.95

FU QING-ZHU'S GYNECOLOGY trans. by Yang Shou-zhong and Liu Da-wei, ISBN 0-936185-35-X, $22.95

FULFILLING THE ESSENCE A Handbook of Traditional & Contemporary Treatments for Female Infertility, by Bob Flaws, ISBN 0-936185-48-1, $19.95

A HANDBOOK OF TRADITIONAL CHINESE DERMATOLOGY by Liang Jian-hui, trans. by Zhang Ting-liang & Bob Flaws, ISBN 0-936185-07-4 $15.95

A HANDBOOK OF TRADITIONAL CHINESE GYNECOLOGY by Zhejiang College of TCM, trans. by Zhang Ting-liang, ISBN 0-936185-06-6 (4nd edit.) $22.95

A HANDBOOK of TCM PEDIATRICS by Bob Flaws, ISBN 0-936185-72-4, $49.95

A HANDBOOK OF TCM UROLOGY & MALE SEXUAL DYSFUNCTION by Anna Lin, OMD, ISBN 0-936185-36-8, $18.95

THE HEART & ESSENCE OF DAN-XI'S METHODS OF TREATMENT by Xu Dan-xi, trans. by Yang Shou-zhong, ISBN 0-926185-49-X, $24.95

HIGHLIGHTS OF ANCIENT ACUPUNCTURE PRESCRIPTIONS trans. by Honora Lee Wolfe & Rose Crescenz ISBN 0-936185-23-6, $14.95

How to Have A HEALTHY PREGNANCY, HEALTHY BIRTH With Traditional Chinese Medicine by Honora Lee Wolfe, ISBN 0-936185-40-6, $9.95

HOW TO WRITE A TCM HERBAL FORMULA: A Logical Methodology for the Formulation & Administration of Chinese Herbal Medicine in Decoction, by Bob Flaws, ISBN 0-936185-49-X, $10.95

IMPERIAL SECRETS OF HEALTH & LONGEVITY by Bob Flaws, ISBN 0-936185-51-1, $9.95

KEEPING YOUR CHILD HEALTHY WITH CHINESE MEDICINE by Bob Flaws, ISBN 0-936185-71-6, $15.95

Li Dong-yuan's TREATISE ON THE SPLEEN & STOMACH, A Translation of the *Pi Wei Lun* by Yang Shou-zhong & Li Jian-yong, ISBN 0-936185-41-4, $22.95

LOW BACK PAIN: Care & Prevention with Traditional Chinese Medicine by Douglas Frank, ISBN 0-936185-66-X, $9.95

MASTER HUA'S CLASSIC OF THE CENTRAL VISCERA by Hua Tuo, ISBN 0-936185-43-0, $21.95

MASTER TONG'S ACUPUNCTURE: An Ancient Lineage for Modern Practice, trans. and commentary by Miriam Lee, OMD, ISBN 0-936185-37-6, $19.95

THE MEDICAL I CHING: Oracle of the Healer Within by Miki Shima, OMD, ISBN 0-936185-38-4, $19.95

MENOPAUSE A Second Spring: Making a Smooth Transition with Traditional Chinese Medicine by

Honora Lee Wolfe ISBN 0-936185-18-X $14.95

MIGRAINES &TRADITIONAL CHINESE MEDICINE: A Layperson's Guide by Bob Flaws ISBN 0-936185-15-5 $11.95

MY SISTER, THE MOON: The Diagnosis & Treatment of Menstrual Diseases by Traditional Chinese Medicine by Bob Flaws, ISBN 0-936185-34-1, $24.95

PAO ZHI: An Introduction to Processing Chinese Medicinals to Enhance Their Therapeutic Effect, by Philippe Sionneau, ISBN 0-936185-62-1, $34.95

PATH OF PREGNANCY, VOL. I, Gestational Disorders by Bob Flaws, ISBN 0-936185-39-2, $19.95

PATH OF PREGNANCY, Vol. II, A Handbook of Trad. Chin. Postpartum Diseases by Bob Flaws. ISBN 0-936185-42-2, $19.95

PEDIATRIC BRONCHITIS: Its Cause, Diagnosis & Treatment According to Traditional Chinese Medicine trans. by Gao Yu-li and Bob Flaws, ISBN 0-936185-26-0 $16.95

PRINCE WEN HUI'S COOK: Chinese Dietary Therapy by Bob Flaws & Honora Lee Wolfe, ISBN 0-912111-05-4, $12.95 (Published by Paradigm Press, Brookline, MA)

THE PULSE CLASSIC: A Translation of the *Mai Jing* by Wang Shu-he, trans. by Yang Shou-zhong ISBN 0-936185-75-9, $54.95